Assessing and Measuring Caring in Nursing and Health Science

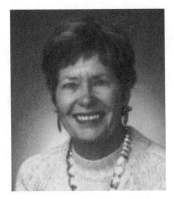 **Jean Watson, PhD, RN, HNC, FAAN,** is Distinguished Professor of Nursing and former Dean of the School of Nursing at the University of Colorado. She is founder of the Center for Human Caring in Colorado, a Fellow of the American Academy of Nursing, and has served as president of the National League for Nursing.

Dr. Watson has earned undergraduate and graduate degrees in nursing and psychiatric-mental health nursing and holds her PhD in educational psychology and counseling. She is a widely published author and recipient of several awards and honors, including an international Kellogg Fellowship in Australia, a Fulbright Research Award in Sweden, and five honorary doctoral degrees, including Honorary International Doctor of Science awards from Goteborg University in Sweden and from Luton University in London.

Clinical nurses and academic programs throughout the world use her published works on the philosophy and theory of human caring and the art and science of caring in nursing. Dr. Watson's caring philosophy is used to guide new models of caring and healing practices in diverse settings worldwide.

At the University of Colorado, Dr. Watson holds the title of Distinguished Professor of Nursing, the highest honor accorded its faculty for scholarly work. In 1998–99 she assumed the nation's first endowed chair in Caring Science, based at the University of Colorado.

Assessing and Measuring Caring in Nursing and Health Science

Jean Watson, RN, PhD, HNC, FAAN

 Springer Publishing Company

Copyright © 2002 by Springer Publishing Company, Inc.

Springer Publishing Company, Inc.
536 Broadway
New York, NY 10012-3955

Acquisitions Editor: Ruth Chasek
Production Editor: Jeanne Libby
Cover design by Susan Hauley

01 02 03 04 05 / 5 4 3 2 1

Library of Congress Cataloging-in-Publication Data

Watson, Jean, 1940–
    Assessing and measuring caring in nursing and health science / Jean Watson.
        p.   cm.
    Includes bibliographical references and index.
    ISBN 0-8261-2313-9
    1. Nursing.   2. Caring.   I. Title.
RT42.W38 2002
610.73—dc21   2001041127
                                                                          CIP

Printed in the United States of America by Sheridan Books

With special tribute to:

KAREN HOLLAND
Former Executive Director
University of Colorado Center for Human Caring
and
JEANNIE ZUK, PhDc
Research Assistant
Doctoral Student Assistant 2000

*With gratitude and recognition to the following
individuals who were doctoral student project
assistants at the University of Colorado
School of Nursing during earlier phases of this project:*

Chantal Cara, PhD
Sharon Cumbie, PhD
Sherry Abbott, MS, PhD student
Dorothy Hughes, PhD
Jean Chow, PhD
Phyllis Eide, PhD
Lizzie Teichler, PhD
Jeannie Zuk, PhDc

Contents

Part III: Challenges and Future Directions

Contributors

Jeannie Zuk, RN, MSN, PhDc
University of Colorado Student
and Doctoral Candidate
University of Colorado Health Sciences Center
School of Nursing
Denver, Colorado

Dr. Carolie Coates, PhD
Research and Measurement Consultant
Boulder, Colorado

Foreword

Nursing is about caring, and when the public thinks about the profession, "caring" often is foremost in their perceptions. What is caring? How do we know it when we see it? What are the vital characteristics of those who care, such as nurses and other health care providers? And most important of all, what difference does caring make in the lives of our clients? This book provides answers and raises issues that are relevant to each of these questions. It not only brings to the forefront the problems and issues in current theories and conceptualizations of caring, but also identifies approaches to the measurement of the concepts which have been derived from multiple perspectives.

This book, which is a compendium of caring instruments, acknowledges the nursing profession's multiple perceptions of caring. Caring may be viewed as an attitude, an ability, an attribute or characteristic, or a complex of interrelated behaviors. The concept is sometimes presented as an adjective, a noun, or a verb in nursing and this book effectively considers measurement approaches that address each of these uses. The author also notes the focus on caring as a process that may be assessed and monitored as an independent variable in research studies, and as a dependent variable or as an outcome itself.

This work brings together into one source the many approaches to conceptualizing caring and the instruments that have been designed to measure it. The author has done a magnificent job in compiling these instruments and providing important information that the reader can use to evaluate their usefulness. When available, questionnaire development procedures, theoretical underpinnings of instruments, reliability and validity of information, and descriptions of instruments and their sources are provided. This book is a reference that will be useful to clinicians, academicians, researchers, nursing care managers, and others who need to select caring instruments for their day-to-day work. It is thought provoking, and a much needed addition to nursing measurement.

Dr. Jean Watson and her colleagues have focused their careers on the phenomenon of caring and this book is another one of their great contributions to the scientific community. The University of Colorado original Center for Human Caring stands as a monument to Dr. Watson's creativity and scholarship and provides a continuing reminder to the world of the centrality of caring to all of us who serve others in the healing professions. Dr. Watson has consistently moved nursing and the scientific community forward through her explorations of the construct of caring. This book is a natural outcome of her work and her focus on caring.

Ora L. Strickland, RN, PhD, FAAN

Preface

The focus of this book is to provide nursing leaders, students, and scholars an up-to-date critique and compilation of the most salient instruments to assess and measure caring. The book is a compendium of instruments available to measure caring, including tools developed, modified, and/or reported in nursing research literature, from 1984 to 2001. It contains an overview of the caring instruments that have been developed by nurse researchers. The measurements help to address quality of care, patient/client/nurse perceptions of caring, caring behaviors, caring abilities, and caring efficacy. The collection encompasses those measurements of caring that have relevance in assessing caring among students as well as patients and nurses, thus allowing use in both educational and clinical care research.

The book offers information on the origin, development, and use of each tool, key citations for the use of each, as well as a copy of the tools themselves. A matrix is provided so the reader can grasp the scope of each measurement, as well as a sense of the total instruments that can be accessed for research use. The matrix protocol includes: conceptual/theoretical orientation relevant to tools development; the author and source citation for tools use; the purpose and/or objectives for the instrument and its use; follow-up revisions, and further development of each instrument, where applicable; participants in use for development and further testing/use of tool; reported reliability and validity of each tool's development; as well as a general description of the instrument, nature of scales, items, and so on. As with use of any instruments, before deciding to use any one of them, it is always appropriate, if not wise, to check for the latest biographical sources for recent updates. With any publication, there is always a time lag and the possibility of changes, revisions, or publication of new versions of the measurement.

During this era of evidence-based practice and outcome demands, the caring instruments in this book can be used as a form of empirical evidence to assist educational and clinical researchers in assessing, if not validating, the critical role of caring and its influence in patient care and outcomes of care practices. It is hoped that these instruments will serve as quality indicators of caring, helping to point nurse researchers toward the deeper human, relational dimensions of caring-based practices.

The instruments may be used as both dependent and independent variables, making their relevance significant and important to clinical research in a time of economic constraints and demand for care/caring, from the public and professionals alike. As such, these caring instruments serve to bridge paradigms between more ethical, theoretical, and philosophical aspects of nurse caring practices, and increasing expectations and accountability for empirical data, to ground the less visible aspects of caring processes and behaviors.

In addition, this collection of 21 caring instruments, taken together, offer a story of nursing theory and knowledge development, as nursing scholars search for, and experiment with, measuring or capturing the elusive phenomena of caring, often considered nonmeasurable. This work stands as a testimony to the nursing scholars who experimented with, and continue to explore, new ways of capturing a core phenomenon of nursing that needs to be made more explicit in both our practices and our outcomes.

The reader will recognize the journey and evolution of the different instruments. You will see how some are theoretically derived and others are a-theoretical in their development; how some have been tested and used across multiple populations and cultures and others are evolving still. This work serves as a tribute to the multiple nursing scholars who have paved the way in this area of caring research, knowledge development, and risk taking.

Lastly, this work may also be considered controversial, in that it is not an answer to the issue of how to capture caring in nursing practice. Rather, the instruments simply serve as indicators along the way, and point back to a deeper dimension of nurses' human caring relational practices, that still remain elusive and non-measurable, as they should be. Nevertheless, empirical indicators that move us closer to recognizing and honoring the deeply human nature of nursing's caring work warrant attention and use in clinical inquiry.

We hope that this collection and critique of the extant caring instruments in the field of nursing will move nursing research and caring knowledge one step forward. This work, thus, seeks to aid nursing in capturing clinical research phenomena through instruments that are sensitive to those practices that nurses and patients hold dear and timeless.

Karen Holland and I, and the doctoral students in the University of Colorado Center for Human Caring, who collectively worked on this project over a five-year period, offer it as a gift to the public that nursing serves, with its long history, if not devotion, to caring. It is our hope that if nursing scholars have greater knowledge and access to instruments to assess and validate caring, new knowledge of caring and nursing science will be forthcoming.

Jean Watson

Acknowledgments

Formal acknowledgments and deep gratitude go to Karen Holland and the staff of the original Center for Human Caring for working with me to birth and sustain this project through various cycles of effort. My continuing appreciation to those doctoral students who committed time and scholarship to the library reviews and searches of these instruments in the literature. More recently I again wish to offer my great appreciation and admiration for the hard work and scholarship of Jeannie Zuk who spent many hours on this project. Her enthusiasm and devotion to scholarship and detective work helped to keep this work alive and current. Dr. Carolie Coates has been a background measurement expert, resource, and critic to me, helping to shape the nature of the critiques and reviews of the instruments. I am appreciative of her willingness to contribute a very important chapter as well as review drafts of earlier sections of the manuscript.

My respect and awe to Charlotte Chin-McMullen for her competence, energy, and salvation in helping to bring this manuscript to completion with her final formatting and ordering of the materials. Finally, I offer my highest respect and thanks to the authors of the tools. We can all be grateful for their pioneering work in caring instruments. I especially appreciate their willingness to be a part of this work. Their feedback and refinements of the text, along with the latest updates on their respective instruments, have helped to make this book as up to date as possible.

Jean Watson
Boulder, Colorado

PART I

Overview

1

Introduction

MEASURING CARING

"What do you mean *measuring caring*? How can you justify having empirical objective measures about such an existential human relational phenomenon as human caring in nursing practice?" These are the questions, silent and spoken, that one hears within nursing circles. Indeed, these are some of my own internal questions which reflect my ambivalence about *measuring caring*. The concern is that in trying to measure caring, one is drawn into a process of reducing a human complex phenomenon down to a level of objectivity that exhausts the deeper meaning.

The very nature of caring, because of its often invisible nature, means that it is considered contradictory to try to reduce it to external, outerworld empirical measures such as a set of behaviors, tasks, or physical-physiological indicators, such as blood pressure or heart rate. The very paradigm in which caring is located, with its ambiguity from the caring theory literature, has tended to make caring almost *un*measurable, both ethically and practically, unless by some qualitative standards that seek to capture the elusive, subjective dimensions.

This dilemma is part of the debate about measuring such a *soft* phenomenon of the human realm. For example, caring is often considered an ontology, a way of being, in contrast to an outward way of doing something that can manifest itself in the physical, external, objective realm.

So, at one end of the continuum, some view caring as a basic motive, a philosophy, an existential intent that cannot be defined in terms of external criteria, but it is "each nurse's own honest attitude to the basic motive" that is important (Lindstrom & Eriksson, 1999). On the other hand there has been a call for nursing to advance its knowledge of caring by advancing "the empirical measurement of caring in a way that withstands the scrutiny of the scientific community" (Valentine, 1991).

An even more complicated aspect of this work, aside from the dialectic debates, or dichotomies, as to how to assess or measure *caring*, is the indistinctness of the concept itself. The common usage of the term *care* belies its complexity (Stockdale & Warelow, 2000). As several authors have noted, *caring* can be an adverb, an adjective, a verb or a noun; it can connote an ontological perspective of being that is often complicated by connotations that define *caring* as *care*, implying the physical, task, external aspect of action or behaviors. These various views of *caring/care* may be, and often are, used interchangeably.

To compound the debate there is the lack of consensus of the place of caring in nursing, due to different conceptualizations of caring. Morse et al. (1991) are often quoted for their identification and critique of at least five views of caring in nursing literature:

- As human trait; as natural condition of being human
- As moral imperative, such as a virtue or value
- An affect, toward oneself, one's patients, one's job
- An interpersonal interaction, something existing between two persons
- A therapeutic intervention, a deliberate act with a planned goal in mind

Other theoretical critiques abound surrounding the concept of caring. Some of the discourse has both questioned and advocated for caring as an ethical, or moral principle; others have opposed viewing caring in any way that may lead to a duty or an obligation; still others have opposed viewing caring in any way that encourages emotional attachment, dependency, inefficiency, and burnout. Nevertheless, it is also noted that caring involves an expression within a personal context calling forth openness, receptiveness, and authenticity. (For further exploration of these points see, Stockdale & Warelow, 2000; Kuhse, 1993; Benner & Wrubel, 1989; Brody, 1988; Fry, 1989; Bowden, 1997; Brown, Kitson, & McKnight, 1992; Watson, 1988; Watson, 1990).

Another dynamic that complicates the location of the concept and phenomenon of caring, within nursing science, includes the metaparadigm debates. Smith (1999) highlights these metaparadigm issues regarding nursing's disciplinary matrix. For example, she noted that while some nursing scholars assert that caring is a central concept in nursing science, others argue that it is ubiquitous, not unique, nonsubstantive, nongeneralizable, feminine, and so on. Others have questioned the use of the term caring in nursing, believing that it is a tautology (Phillips, 1993).

These opposing points of view about the meaning and placement of caring, within nursing science and its disciplinary knowledge domain, have led to dualistic views of measuring caring. The end result has been tension around methodologies, resulting in schisms between qualitative and quantitative approaches to nursing phenomena in general, and caring phenomena in particular.

There still remain some lingering questions around nursing's epistemologies; they are leaning toward the empirical during this time of management, control of costs, and care. Often these new management-generated activities around care are determined by medical, economic, and administrative considerations, rather than caring needs and process from patients' and nurses' perspectives. Administrative, operational, and economic motivations often dominate. By having access to nursing-sensitive indicators of care/caring that many of the caring instruments represent, researchers and administrators alike can come closer to sustaining a caring orientation in the midst of health care reforms. By assessing caring empirically, nursing and other health sciences may uncover more of a caring science view about its basic, relational/ontological assumptions. In addition by researching caring formally, the conceptual/theoretical caring philosophies may more clearly emerge, thereby more clearly informing the biophysical/technological model of care.

There are still rhetorical questions about nursing's tendency to jump to methods and models of measurement before addressing the meaningful, philosophical questions that inform both method and measurement. While these questions and debate will continue, this collection of caring instruments is a means to bridge debates and dualisms, and paradigms. Researching caring does not guarantee caring ideology, attitudes, and manifestations in practice, but leads closer to putting caring into the formula.

Empirical studies of caring show that nurses recognize, and take into consideration, the patient's caring needs on the basis of the prevalent caring culture (Fagerstrom & Engberg, 1998). By having instruments to address caring, there are more possibilities for developing knowledge of caring, and learning more about how patients, nurses, and systems may benefit.

Moreover, it is a time to open to an era of shifting and emergent paradigms, of moving between worldviews and dualistic opposites; it is a time for openness, for exploration, a time of pragmatics, and heuristic means to move forward. Contemporary dualistic debates and mindsets about caring in nursing science will probably not go away. However, it is a moment in nursing's history to reconcile dualisms and either/or positions, whether they be about caring/noncaring in the disciplinary matrix, or about measuring/nonmeasuring views of caring in nursing.

Compromises can and are made, and assumptions can be purposefully violated, if one can remain mindful and conscious about what compromises are made, and when they are made, and for what goals. This work acknowledges that some deep philosophical/ontological dimensions of caring cannot be measured, but some measurement can elucidate the manifest field of caring practice, while still pointing toward the nonmanifest whole.

In addition, it is important to honor human caring as having a central and significant place in nursing science, in that caring offers a values foundation for the profession, as well as a ground for additional knowledge to guide clinical practice and research. The whole realm of human relationships, health, and healing may be tied back to caring as the basis of the relationship. Thus the ability to capture the phenomenon of caring, and its affect on health and healing, may provide new knowledge and insights about practice. Caring-based models may indeed be detected that affect both costs and outcomes, as well as improve working environments for practitioners and patients alike.

Once some aspects of these deep positions and debates are acknowledged they open up a horizon of possibilities that can be informed by the dialectical dance, rather than polarized in an either/or position. While caring may never be truly measured, this collection of extant measurement instruments is one means toward a partial end of assessing and capturing the phenomena of caring and its relationship to patient outcomes. If more evidence can be offered, in the form of quality indicators of caring, then nursing is positioned to manifest more clearly that which is often taken for granted or dismissed. In addition, empirical evidence of caring, captured in an elusive practice world that is unstable, unseen, chaotic, and changing, can be a tangible grasp and glimpse of nursing's contribution to both science, and public health and welfare.

Caring, once glimpsed through empirical measures, whether they be qualitative or quantitative, may help us to see what has been long hidden from our public consciousness as well as our science. More specifically, the purposes for the use of formal measurement tools in nursing research on caring include:

- Continuous improvement of caring by using outcomes to improve practices through more mindful interventions
- Benchmarking structures and settings whereby caring is more manifest
- Tracking of levels and models of caring in care settings against routine care practices
- Evaluating consequences of caring vs. noncaring for both nurses and patients
- Creating a "report card" model of a unit or an institution in a critical area of practice
- Identifying areas of weakness and strength in caring processes and interventions in order to stimulate self-correction and models of excellence in practice

- Increasing our knowledge and understanding between caring relationships and health and healing
- Empirically validating extant caring theories, as well as generating new theories of caring, caring relationships, and health practices
- Stimulating new directions for nursing, caring, and health sciences, including interdisciplinary/transdisciplinary research

Measuring caring? Yes, this work offers multiple means to measure caring, while still knowing that any measurement is only a manifestation, an indicator of something deeper. The "something deeper" remains in the world of human and caring science phenomena that may never be fully known, but indicated. These instruments serve as pointers along the way.

The measurement tools of caring included in this work have not developed in any particular systematic way, but rather through the interest of individuals, with some being informed by specific theories of caring. While different theories of caring have stimulated nursing research on the phenomena of caring itself, in some other instances these theories have stimulated development of specific tools for assessing caring. Some of the measurement tools here have evolved a priori to capture significant indicators of caring, based on general information and the literature of both nursing and related fields, such as psychology and philosophy. Others have been devised from certain implicit philosophical assumptions about what caring is; thus, there is a connection between the choice of the caring measures to be assessed and the prevailing philosophy of caring.

Taken together, they represent the major measurements tools on caring that have been reported in the nursing literature since the early 1980s (Larson et al., 1984) through the latest instruments developed and published in 1999–2000 (Arthur, 1999; Coates, 1999; Shepherd & Sherwood, 2000; Swanson, 2000). This work offers a matrix structure and framework for all these tools. The matrix includes the following information:

- Identity of each of the measurements when developed
- The author(s) and contact information
- The year published and key source citation(s) in literature
- What the tool was developed to measure
- A description of the instrument
- The nature and number of participants in tool development
- Reported reliability/validity, if available
- Whether the theory is derived or a-theoretical (conceptual basis of measure)
- Latest citations for instrument use in nursing literature

In addition to the matrix format for each of the caring measurement tools, each of the instruments is included in the appendix along with information as to specific requirements for its use.

This collection, and this compilation of measurements of caring, offer a foundation for furthering the field of caring research. However, for nursing science to move forward in the area of quality, outcomes, and evidence, along with relationships between caring-based interventions and costs, new instruments and processes will have to develop and evolve. The future may lead to the use of hard science criteria, and even the possibility of biological instrumentation, to capture a soft science experience and expression such as human caring. New insights and greater depths of construct validity will be of importance as this work is further developed. It is anticipated that even more sophistication in next-generation design, method, measurement, and analysis of data will increase in precision and allow the creative emergence of new options (Smith & Reeder, 1998).

RECONCILING NURSING THEORY AND ONTOLOGICAL/ METHODOLOGICAL CONGRUENCE FOR MEASURING CARING

In measuring caring, it is proposed that one can do so in such a way that honors, advances, and even violates some assumptions about caring and measuring caring. It is within this debate, this dialectic, that compromises are mindfully made, with the hope that in mindfully measuring caring, nursing science and knowledge moves forward within its own unique framework for clinical nursing research, evidence, and outcomes. As Smith and Reeder (1998) suggest, there are ways to reconcile conceptual inconsistencies between methodology, epistemology, and ontology within a nursing science context. For example, in their research on Therapeutic Touch (TT) they adhered to Rogerian Science (1970), and a framework of Unitary Human Being. In doing so, they reconciled inconsistencies between traditional and Rogerian Science by honoring that therapeutic touch encompasses the caring intention of the practitioner and rhythmic movement as essential processes of touch therapies; therefore, that was one way of "participating in the dynamic flow of the human/environment field patterning . . . that healing may be reflected in multiple manifestations of patterning, from physical, even cellular changes, to perception, images, and shifts in awareness . . . that caring intention and rhythmic movement potentiate pattern change; and this pattern change . . . may be evident in multiple field manifestations . . . " (Smith & Reeder, 1998).

Such reconciliation and logical deduction from the paradigm or theoretical level, to relational statements, can be made in a similar way in seeking to "measure caring." For example, moving from caring theory at the meta-level to empirical measures, one can highlight linkages between theory, measurement, and selected outcomes. Since most of the measurement tools in this book were developed from theories and/or were derived from conceptual systems, it is anticipated that new measures will continue to evolve that will offer closer ontological/methodological congruency, and/ or make overt where any reconciliation is made.

Each conceptual/theoretical system of caring used to inform the developments of the different tools could be traced back to implied philosophical assumptions, as well as middle-range theory, practice, or research tradition related to each of them. The research traditions are the "designs, methods, data forms, and analytic processes that best help the scientist develop and test the middle range theories emerging from the broader grand theory or conceptual model" (Smith & Reeder, 1998). Here we can acknowledge that a context for research and use of measurement for the phenomenon of caring, holds within it the foundational ontological and epistemological assumptions implied or made explicit; while those assumptions inform design, methods, and data forms for a study, the "ontological paradigms within the discipline may be consistent with more than one epistemic paradigm" (Smith & Reeder, 1998), allowing for both existing and newly developed instruments, data forms, and combinations of qualitative and quantitative data that best capture the complexities of the nature and quality of human caring. Measuring caring within this context takes on a different meaning and may allow researchers to be more explicit that the empirical tools make manifest key indicators of caring, while honoring the nonmanifest field that is emerging and unseen behind the empirics. Reminding ourselves that the empirics of caring measurements are not the phenomenon itself, but only an indicator. The empirical indicators cannot be understood alone by themselves, but must be relocated back into the conceptual system or model from which they were derived. In other words, the parts that become objectively present in the "manifest field" must be placed within the context of the whole from which they emerged. The findings can then be interpreted/reinterpreted within the theoretical/ conceptual context, and not stand alone as "isolated evidence." It is through such efforts to connect research traditions, designs, methods, measurements, and insights, and findings that new insights, theories, and research can be generated. As a result, new insights and evidence can be obtained and both shortcomings as well as strengths of existing tools can be identified, paving the way for a new generation of measurements and design as well as theory evolution.

In summary: Measuring caring? Yes, but intentionally and mindfully, with a consciousness that deep caring cannot be fully "measured" at this time. At best these measurements serve as quality empirical indicators of caring and point back toward the deeper aspects behind the measurements. Nevertheless, just because caring is a complex human phenomenon does not mean we should not try to capture as much of the depth of the phenomenon as possible. In doing so, clarification of assumptions can be made, and reconciliation identified between ontological, epistemological assumptions within the various theoretical/conceptual system of caring. Finally, the result may lead to better fits between and among research traditions, design methods, and the processes used for creative emergence: the use of extant, as well as new, forms of caring inquiry.

2

Caring and Nursing Science: Contemporary Discourse

STATE OF CARING KNOWLEDGE IN NURSING SCIENCE

In addition to the debate about measuring caring, and the ambiguity around the concept itself, there also is uncertainty about the state of caring knowledge in nursing. While there is a lack of consensus about the nature of caring, as well as its location within nursing's disciplinary matrix, it seems clear that further development of the knowledge of caring is one seminal aspect of nursing's distinction. Indeed, while the academic debates may linger, clinical care issues accelerate, and the demand for nursing practices that sustain caring become more critical than ever. Therefore, it is important to point out some of the converging developments that position caring and caring knowledge more clearly within nursing's domain of concern.

One attempt to reconcile the dissonance around caring in nursing was the Newman, Sime, and Corcoran-Perry (1991) critique of the existing metaparadigm. They noted the need for more explicit connectedness and social relevance to describe the field of study. They asserted that caring and health are linked within theoretical literature in nursing; that the quality of the relationship is what facilitates health and makes it possible for nurse and patient to connect in a way that is transforming. Thus they presented a unifying statement for the disciplinary focus by framing nursing as "the study of caring in the human health experience" (Newman et al., 1991).

Smith (1999) also has made a strong case for the concept of caring, critiquing and then offering counterpoints to arguments for why caring is not a central concept. For example, she made the case that none of the concerns for not including caring hold merit, overturning arguments relating to ambiguity, limiting perspective, ubiquitous, non-substantive, nongeneralizable, and feminine. She went on to identify five constitutive meanings of caring from the perspective of Rogerian science of Unitary Human Beings: (1) manifesting intentions; (2) appreciating pattern; (3) attuning to dynamic flow; (4) experiencing the infinite; and (5) inviting creative emergence (Smith, 1999).

Each of these constitutive meanings are present in extant nursing literature. Smith explicated semantic expressions of each of these meanings. A modified version of her summaries is included here in tables 1–5 (Smith, 1999).

In spite of a lack of formal disciplinary consensus about caring as part of the metaparadigm of nursing, caring has emerged during the past three decades as a central component and paradigm of nursing. Newman et al. (1991), Smith (1999), and others (Watson & Smith, 2000) help to make this explicit and a valid fact at this point in time.

RECENT DISCIPLINARY DIRECTIONS AFFIRMING "CARING" IN NURSING

In addition to the above developments, some other major events attest to the centrality of caring as part of nursing's focus. For example, the following evidence has accumulated in the past few years, attesting to the relevance and presence of caring knowledge as a focus in nursing:

TABLE 2.1 Expression of Caring: Manifesting Intention

Semantic expression of nurse caring: manifesting intentions

Person-centered intention
Preserving dignity and humanity
Committed to alleviating vulnerability
Giving attention and concern
Reverence for person and human life
Love and co-presence
Authenticity and availability
Being with
Attention, compassion, focus
Feeling compassion
Regard
Intentional presence
Being with the other
Intention of knowing, acknowledging, affirming, celebrating the other

Diverse sources in nursing literature (modified from Smith, 1999).

TABLE 2.2   Expressions of Caring: Appreciating Pattern

Semantic expressions of caring: appreciating pattern

Placing value on the other as lovable, worthy of being loved
Cherishing the wholeness of the human being
Assuming the subjectivity of the other as valid and whole
Acknowledging the emerging pattern without trying to change it
Confirming of human dignity
Seeing the other as perfect in the moment
Unfolding possibilities for becoming
Yearning for a deeper understanding and appreciation of the natural healing
   resources
Life force, pattern, and paradox
Sensitivity to pattern manifestations that give identify to each unique person
Transcending judgment
Seeing underneath fragmentation to existence of wholeness

Diverse sources in nursing literature (modified from Smith, 1999).

TABLE 2.3   Expression of Caring: Attuning to Dynamic Flow

Semantic expressions of nurse caring: attuning to dynamic flow

Attuned to subtleties in the moment
Sensitivity to self and other
Connected
Belonging and interconnected
Living in context of relational
Detecting the person's being and feeling the condition
Synchronization and organismic integration
Action of love
Energetic resonance
Pattern or vibration of nurse's consciousness becoming attuned with other

Diverse sources in nursing literature (modified from Smith, 1999).

- Academic nursing structures and academic departments in Scandinavian countries named "Caring Science"
- Two international journals in nursing with focus on caring: *Scandinavian Journal of Caring Science,* and *International Journal of Human Caring*
- International Professional Nursing Organization International Association of Human Caring (IAHC)—21 years old
- "Caring Science" *The Science of Caring* research publications (University of California, San Francisco)—12 years

TABLE 2.4   Expressions of Caring: Experiencing the Infinite

Semantic expression of caring: experiencing the infinite

Transcends physical and material world, bound in time and space
Expanded sense of self: transcendent qualities
Highest form of knowing
Unfolding divine love
Ontological mystery
Spiritual union—transcending self, time, and space
Spirit of both present, expands the limits of openness
Caring moment relations between past/present and imagined future

Diverse sources in nursing literature (modified from Smith, 1999).

TABLE 2.5   Expressions of Caring: Inviting Creative Emergence

Semantic expression of caring: inviting creative emergence

Holding hopeful orientation
Growing in capacity to express caring
Transforming mutual process
Caring action; growth of spiritual life within
Calling to deeper life; birthing spiritual life in each person
Expanding human capacities
Facilitating creative emergence

Diverse sources in nursing literature (modified from Smith, 1999).

- Key recommendations for caring as core concept in nursing—National reports: American Academy Nursing (AAN) Wingspread Conference
- National League for Nursing (NLN) curriculum standards
- Special devoted monographs, conferences, journal issues on caring
- American Nurses Association (ANA) revised Definition-Social Policy Statement with inclusion of caring and caring relationships as new definition (1995)
- Ethical and clinical consequences of Caring/Noncaring (Halldorsdottir, 1999)
- Metaanalysis of 130 empirical nursing studies (Swanson, 1999).

This accumulation of converging developments helps to resolve the dissonance about caring and its place in nursing science. Whether one considers the issues as an unresolved discourse, or whether one considers caring as a central or unifying concept for the discipline, the need to grasp the phenomenon in diverse ways is one of the responsibilities for nursing's maturity.

MEASURING CARING AND OUTCOMES—NURSING KNOWLEDGE AND INTERNATIONAL RESEARCH PRIORITIES

Hinshaw's recent review of trends in nursing knowledge pointed out Sigma Theta Tau International's Strategic Plan for 2005: "To create a global community of nurses who lead in using scholarship, knowledge, and technology to improve the health of the world's people" (Hinshaw, 2000).

As part of her review Hinshaw provided three perspectives for generating nursing knowledge trends and identified priorities for the 21st century:

- Via an analysis of the top five nursing research priorities evident in the American nursing literature of past 5 years
- Via future directions for nursing research outlined by 60 American investigators
- Via identified international nursing research priorities from a number of countries.

Related to the discussion here on issues about measurement of caring, it is interesting to note from Hinshaw's review that priority areas, identified by both American nursing scholars and relevant U.S. nursing publications, include "quality of care outcomes and their measurements, impact or effectiveness of nursing interventions." In other words, as Hinshaw noted, "The emphasis on quality of care outcomes indicates the profession's commitment to identify and measure nursing-sensitive outcomes as both clinical measures and research tools."

What is perhaps even more interesting than the general consensus within American nursing research priorities, is the fact that similar priorities relating to concern for care issues, quality of care outcomes, and nursing interventions are identified in international nursing circles. For example, in Great Britain "research into patients' perspectives of care and how they are assessed," and "nursing interventions" were named as priorities; in the Nordic countries "quality of care balanced with cost outcomes," along with theoretical and philosophical perspectives of developing knowledge in nursing practice" were identified as their top issues; in Thailand and Africa priorities for nursing research included "improvement of nursing interventions" and "care of individuals" with specific conditions. Similarly, The European Work Group, representing 19 European countries, included "effective care and continuity (of care across settings)" and "effect of variations . . . on quality and costs of care and patient outcomes" in their challenges for generating knowledge for the discipline of nursing (Hinshaw, 2000).

What is dramatic is the fact that in all of these international nursing circles, care issues and outcomes of care, along with measurement of both, loomed as the top priorities for nursing research. Hence, a collection of tools or measurements of caring, as indicators of nursing-sensitive approaches to these global nursing priorities, is relevant to the facilitation of further knowledge and research. Researching the phenomenon of caring more specifically and intentionally within the context of "quality of caring outcomes" as well as "impact or effectiveness of nursing interventions" can help inform and strengthen both the discipline and the practice of nursing for the 21st century.

EMPIRICAL OUTCOMES OF CARING RESEARCH: CONSEQUENCES OF CARING/NONCARING IN NURSING

While Smith and others have made a theoretical and philosophical case for caring within nursing, the above discussion highlights broader international professional activities, priorities, structures, organizations, position statements, definitions, and so forth. Taken together, these intellectual and professional developments attest to the placement of caring within the discipline and priorities for researching and measuring care/caring and its outcomes as almost a universal mandate in nursing circles.

However, even more convincing perhaps is the recent work in the empirical domain itself. Swanson's (1999) review and meta-analysis of 130 empirical nursing research studies offer further evidence as to the importance of caring and its outcomes; indeed, it helps to reveal both consequences of caring and noncaring for both patients and nurses.

For example, Tables 2.6 and 2.7 summarize the empirical findings with respect to outcomes and consequences of caring vs. noncaring, and the effects of caring vs. noncaring on both patients and nurses.

These conclusions and findings from Swanson's meta-analysis of a range of empirical studies of caring in nursing science literature offer important information, attesting to the continued importance of creating both structures and processes whereby caring can occur between nurses and patients. The consequences of both caring and noncaring for nurses and patients are dramatic messages for nursing research and practice.

At a time when nursing is declining and its survival threatened, nurses' satisfaction is enhanced when caring is able to be practiced. When caring

TABLE 2.6   Empirical Outcomes of Caring Research: Patients

Consequences of Caring Research Outcomes of Caring for Patients (Summary of Findings)	Consequences of Noncaring Research Outcomes of Noncaring for Patients (Summary of Findings)
• Emotional/spiritual well-being (dignity, self-control, personhood) • Physical enhanced healing, lives saved, safety, more energy, fewer costs, more comfort, less loss • Trust relationship, decrease in alienation, closer family relations	• Humiliated, frightened, out of control, despair, helplessness, alienation, vulnerability, lingering bad memories • Decreased healing

(Based upon meta-analysis of 130 empirical studies, Swanson, 1999)

TABLE 2.7   Empirical Outcomes of Caring Research: Nurses

Consequences of Caring Research Outcomes of Caring for Nurses (Summary of Findings)	Consequences of Noncaring Research Outcomes of Noncaring for Nurses (Summary of Findings)
• Emotional/spiritual—sense of accomplishment, satisfaction, purpose, gratitude • Preserved integrity, fulfillment, wholeness, self-esteem • Living own philosophy • Respect for life, death • Reflective • Love of nursing, increased knowledge	• Hardened • Oblivious • Depressed • Frightened • Worn down

(Based upon meta-analysis of 130 empirical studies, Swanson, 1999)

is not present in nursing practices or settings, research indicates that nurses become depressed, robotic, hardened, oblivious, and worn down. This empirical data invites much more research and attention to explore emotional and physical healing consequences for patients when caring is present, including cost savings. The same is true from the other side of the equation, in that nurses are much more satisfied, fulfilled, more purposeful, and knowledge seeking when caring is present.

The instruments that have been developed to empirically assess caring offer one pathway toward more focused research. When evidence of caring is made more manifest it can then be explored more systematically for models of practice excellence. By continuing to explore the phenomenon of caring, through empirical measures, as well as non-empirical means, nursing continues to build its *nursing* science foundation for a new century of nursing practice.

The importance of developing and researching caring knowledge and practices within nursing science has another contribution to make at this turn in nursing's history. For example, nursing scholars have addressed the unsettled state of nursing knowledge. As recently as 1999 Fawcett noted "a very real concern for the continued existence of the discipline of nursing . . . " (Fawcett, 1999). In critiquing the hallmarks of 20th and 21st century nursing theory and knowledge development, she acknowledged some major highlights of accomplishment:

• Specification of metaparadigm for nursing knowledge
• Explication of conceptual models
• Explication of unique nursing theories
• Theories shared with other disciplines.

In spite of these accomplishments, she and others such as Kim (1996) suggest that issues of fragmentation, arbitrariness and lack of nursing research that truly advances *nursing* science (in contrast to other disciplines and medical science), are all lingering dilemmas for nursing to resolve, if it is to survive as a distinct discipline and mature profession. By more specifically attending to, and researching the caring phenomena in nursing practice, as both process and outcomes, as well as considering the caring relationship as part of the nature of specific intervention models for practice, nursing knowledge is generated that can contribute to strengthening the distinct nature of nursing's role and importance in clinical care.

However, nursing is not alone in identifying care issues and outcomes. Indeed, other disciplines now also are recognizing and incorporating caring into their disciplinary foci, for example:

• Caring/therapeutics, in health practices in general, is occurring among a range of diverse practitioners
• Relationship-centered care/caring as a major initiative among health care reform recommendations (e.g., Fetzer Institute project on Relationship-Centered Care)
• Feminist studies
• Women's health
• Ethics
• Philosophy

- Emergence of caring science as entity in its own right (Eriksson & Lindstrom, 1999).

Indeed, in the field of medicine some empirical research findings relating to caring relationships and communication between physicians and patients reinforce the empirical findings of Swanson's (1999) analysis in the nursing science field. Frankel (1994) found that the relationship between patient and physician and the nature of the communication was related to both formal and informal complaints and litigation from patients. A link was found between the absence of a caring relationship, patient dissatisfaction, and depositions of lawsuits. Such convergence of outcomes of caring research, in both nursing science and medical research, attest to the importance of more research in the field, and the need for access to empirical indicators for measuring caring. Nursing science and nursing researchers offer an array of empirical measurements as a background and foundation for additional nursing and interdisciplinary research on caring outcomes, as well as a basis for addressing care/caring measurements issues.

3

Background for Selection of Caring Instruments

Jean Watson and Jeannie Zuk

This project began approximately six years ago as an initiative in the Center for Human Caring at the University of Colorado under the guidance of the then Center Director, Dr. Jean Watson. The project had the special administration leadership of Karen Holland, the Executive Director of the Center. Due to some life changes of Dr. Watson and system/administrative changes, the project was interrupted between 1997 and 1999. It was reactivated in 1999 with the special research and tracking skill assistance of Jeannie Zuk, PHDc, a doctoral student and research assistant in the University of Colorado School of Nursing. Over these past few years there have been a cadre of devoted University of Colorado doctoral nursing students who engaged in intensive research to identify and update the development and use of any empirical measurement tools of caring (Assistants are listed on the dedication page).

To initiate the original project, an extensive review of the CINAHL database was conducted to identify all empirical caring measurements that were published in the nursing literature. Once initiated, each doctoral student cohort engaged in intensive, and extensive, follow-up of the use of the specific measurements, as well as locating the origin and name of the tool's developer, and other studies that used the measurement. The earliest one detected was published by Larson (1984).

When the study was reactivated in 1999, the original CINAHL search was used as a basis for updating the instrument matrix. Two other databases were used to expand the search: Health & Psychosocial Instruments and

MEDLINE. Each of the originally identified tools was entered into all three databases to find both primary and secondary references to the tools. Serendipity led to what proved to be a key article in identifying new instruments (Beck, 1999), and an additional six instruments were added to the matrix. Each of the 16 tools was then entered into each of the three databases and the search took on the characteristics of a detective pursuing a case. The references listed in published articles were tracked down as leads or contacts with authors. The Internet was useful in finding current addresses for authors.

The search for each of these tools and their additional use has continued through diverse approaches. Once additional studies were located, there was follow-up with key words. Terms such as caring, care, measurement, tool, instrument, as well as the names of specific instruments were used. A range of empirical measurements emerged that included caring attributes, caring behaviors, patients' perception, and satisfaction with nurses' caring. As a result of the diversity of approaches, caring is treated in different ways and there are varying conceptual notions that underlie their developments. Likewise, there are varying degrees of reliability and validity. The measurements included here all have some reports of reliability and validity, and there is an attempt to note the conceptual/theoretical origin of the instruments development. There is no attempt to do an extensive psychometric critique of each instrument. Rather, we have attempted to report the face value of each of the measurements, some of the major background facts about its development, and the source citations for research using the tool.

The search for publication citations as well as author contact, continued through January 2001. Where possible, each author was contacted, with an invitation to review the information that was developed; each had the opportunity to offer any corrections, updates, revisions, and so on. It was most helpful to have information and responses from the individual authors to make the material as accurate and current as possible.

Final compilation of each measurement, and its update, resulted in the final matrix which includes:

- Instrument, year developed
- Author(s), developers, and contact address
- Publication source citation title; journal and year published
- What each tool was developed to measure
- A description of the instrument
- Participants (sample) in research and development
- Reported reliability and validity
- Conceptual/theoretical origin
- The latest citation for the tool found in nursing literature.

The result includes a review of all studies and citations of caring measurements that were reported between 1984 and 2001. Multiple citations were discovered that addressed "measuring caring" or cited the use of some instrument to assess caring. In addition, 21 instruments were identified as specific, separate tools for the formal, empirical "measurement" of caring.

A comprehensive blueprint, in the form of a master matrix, found at the end of the book, provides an overview of the nature and status of the all the instruments. The following sections present a summary of specific measurements, and an individual matrix for each instrument, which provides an overview of key characteristics. To the best of my knowledge, the ordering of the instruments is chronological. In some instances there is ambiguity as to which instruments may have been developed first, due to date of publication, even though developmental efforts occurred prior to publication. The date of publication was the date selected for chronological ordering, although earlier developmental dates were noted in the summary and matrix of the specific instruments, when available.

While the final section of the book includes a comprehensive matrix of all the instruments, individual instruments themselves are included in the chapter devoted to its discussion. This is done with permission from the authors and/or publishers of the instruments. The blueprint matrix, combined with selected copies of the measurements themselves, make this book a handy resource for anyone wishing to obtain information, summary data, and access to empirical instruments that measure caring.

PART II

Summary of Each Instrument for Measuring Caring

4

CARE-Q and CARE/SAT

(Larson, 1984, Larson and Ferketich, 1993)

SUMMARY

The Caring Assessment Report Evaluation Q-sort, commonly known as CARE-Q (Larson, 1984), was the first quantitative caring tool cited in the nursing literature, and the most frequently used instrument for assessing caring. It has the longest reputation for repeated use and has generated additional empirical research, in different settings, with different patient populations, as well as generating cross-cultural versions of the tool. More recently, Larson and Ferketich (1993) refined the CARE-Q into a caring satisfaction instrument (CARE/SAT) to attempt to measure patient satisfaction with the nursing care received.

The original tool was developed from somewhat of an a priori orientation to care/caring assumptions, acknowledging some of the early writers in the field of caring theory and philosophies at the time, but the CARE-Q items were developed from the ground up with special concern about the caring needs and perceptions of cancer patients. The view of nurse caring used to inform the instrument's development was "intent to create a subjective sense of feeling cared for in the patient. Feeling cared for is a sensation of well-being and safety resulting from enacted behaviors of another" (Larson, 1986). The specified intent of the instrument is to measure, by ranked importance, the differences and similarities of perceptions that nurses and patients have of identified nurse caring behaviors.

In developing the tool itself, Larson used a Delphi survey of practicing nurses on caring behaviors, and a study of patients' perceptions of nurse caring behaviors which resulted in the identification of 69 nurse caring behaviors, which later was reduced to fifty items, each printed on an individual card. The 50 behavioral items were then ordered in six subscales of caring which include: accessible (six items); comforts (nine items); anticipates (five items); trusting relationship (16 items); monitors and follows through (eight items).

The first generation, as well as later versions of the instrument, used a Q-methodology to identify the most important, nurse caring behaviors as perceived by patients. With this methodology only a certain number of cards can be placed within each designated pile. Thus, each participant is faced with a forced-choice distribution. A predetermined number of items are to be selected in each of the categories from most important to least important. Once the items are selected with the forced choice format, the CARE-Q sort of each participant is then numerically coded for statistical analysis.

An expert nurse panel of graduate nursing students and faculty, who agreed upon 60 items, established the content validity. A panel of nurses and patients on an oncology unit verified these items. As a result, the final version of CARE-Q comprised 50 agreed upon items and six evolved themes. Larson (1987) then attempted to establish reliability and validity. Face and content validity were identified from a sample of both nurses and patients. The test-retest reliability of the CARE-Q was obtained from a sample of 82 randomly selected national oncology nurses (from a national oncology organization). The most important caring items have a test-retest reliability of 79%, and for the least important caring items the result was 63% (Beck, 1999; Andrews, Daniels, & Hall, 1996; Kyle, 1995).

Larson (1984, 1986) identified some limitations of the Q-methodology and the forced choice format of the CARE-Q. The forced choice format has led to difficulties in selecting one item over another as the most important; others commented they would have liked to respond a second time to the selection; others reported that they wished they had done the Q-sort the way they wanted to, as opposed to the way they felt they should (Kyle, 1995). Other critiques include the length of time to complete the CARE-Q (reported to be 26 minutes), and problems related to the fact that some participants did not sort the cards according to directions (Beck, 1999). Kyle notes these shortcomings and raises the question as to the validity of the instrument.

In spite of limitations, numerous other studies have reported use of the original CARE-Q or culturally derived versions of it. Beck (1999) identified several studies that report reliabilities for the CARE-Q, which are described in Table 4.1 below.

To date, no new reliability or validity work on the CARE-Q has been found to occur. Aside from those studies cited above by Beck (1999),

TABLE 4.1   Studies/Reliabilities of CARE-Q

Study	Sample	Reliability
Komorita et al. (1991)	110 master's prepared nurses	*Test-retest reliability* 64.4% for five most important and five least important caring behaviors with 9 nurses
Gooding et al. (1993)	42 oncology patients	+1.00 with 9 nursing students and 46 nurses in Canada
Scharf & Caley (1993)	80 nurses, 50 coronary care patients, and 321 physicians	70% for five most important and 88% for five least important caring items with 10 physicians
Von Essen & Sjoden (1991)	86 medical-surgical patients and 73 nursing staff in Sweden	*Internal Consistency* Total Cronbach's alpha = 0.95. Subscales: • explains and facilitates = 0.59 • comforts = 0.86 • trusting relationship = 0.86 • anticipates = 0.72 • monitors and follows through = 0.79 • accessible = 0.76
Widmark-Patersson et al. (1996)	72 cancer patients and 63 nurses	Total Cronbach's alpha = 0.94 Subscales: • explains and facilitates = 0.60 • comforts = 0.78 • trusting relationship = 0.86 • anticipates = 0.60 • monitors and follows through = 0.59 • accessible = 0.59

researchers have relied largely upon Larson's original tool developmental work. This remains the case although other researchers using the tool noted some of the problems in its use, e.g., nonspecific and vague items leading to a variety of interpretations; length and time to complete, and difficulty in understanding all of the instrument statements (Kyle, 1995).

Nevertheless, studies using the CARE-Q instrument have found agreement on the most important ranked caring behaviors perceived by nurses and patients; however, there is a difference reported between the patients' perceptions of caring and those of nurses, with nurses focusing on psychosocial skills, and patient focusing on those skills which demonstrate professional competency (Kyle, 1995). Various interpretations of these finding have been attempted, with no resolution of these differences, even with additional research and new explanatory models. As a result of these original findings of perceptual differences between nurses and patients, the CARE-Q has stimulated additional research and continuing use up to the present.

Further testing of psychometric properties of this instrument, with some attention to the length and ambiguity of the sorting process and the possibility of constructing a Likert format to make CARE-Q more user friendly (Andrews, Daniels, & Hall, 1996) are recommended for the next generation. Further refinement and evolution of this important, widely used empirical measurement of caring is necessary to strengthen the reliability of the findings with ease of use. The matrix which follows includes background information on the original CARE-Q, along with all the research studies that have been generated using the CARE-Q, including two cultural versions: Swedish and Chinese. Before the formal matrix there is a brief, summary discussion of a recently developed questionnaire that is based on the original CARE-Q, the Care Satisfaction Questionnaire (CARE/SAT) (Larson & Ferketich, 1993).

CARE SATISFACTION QUESTIONNAIRE (CARE/SAT)

This scale was developed by Larson and Ferketich (1993) as an extension of the CARE-Q. They incorporated all 50 items of the CARE-Q into a visual analogue scale (VAS) and renamed it the CARE Satisfaction Questionnaire (CARE/SAT). Some additional items were developed and added in order to assess overall patient satisfaction with nurse caring behaviors. It was finalized to consist of 29 behaviors. The initial testing of the CARE/SAT included 268 hospitalized adult medical-surgical patients ready for discharge within a 48-hour period. Cronbach's alpha for the total scale was reported as 0.94. The authors reported a Pearson correlation coefficient ($r = 0.80$) between the CARE/SAT and the Risser Patient Questionnaire (Hinshaw & Atwood, 1982). This correlation provided evidence of construct validity.

Limited use of this instrument has occurred to date. Some of the difficulties are related to negatively worded statements mixed with those positively worded. Each patient is asked to place an "X" on a 100 mm visual analog line, according to the degree of agreement or disagreement. Because the behaviors are worded both positively and negatively is has been reported as difficult and tedious to analyze, also suggesting that total scores are unreliable for use in a correlation design study (Andrews, Daniels, & Hall, 1996). This instrument is in its first generation of development and use. However, in the Andrew's et al. (1996) discussion, it was reported that the CARE/SAT had one of the shortest mean times to complete (6 minutes) and that the instrument specifically addressed caring actions and perceived caring as a therapeutic intervention.

TABLE 4.2 Matrix of Care-Q and CARE/SAT

Instrument	Author Contact Address	Publication Citation Source	Developed to Measure	Instrument Description	Participants	Reported Validity/ Reliability	Conceptual/ Theoretical Basis of Measurement	Latest Citation in Nursing Literature
Caring Assessment Instrument (CARE-Q) 1984	Patricia Larson, RN, DNS (Retired from) Univ. of California, San Francisco (UCSF) School of Nursing Department of Physiology Nursing Box 0610 N 611Y San Francisco, CA 94143-0610 *pattwkw@ msn.com*	Larson, P. (1984). Important nurse caring behaviors perceived by patients with cancer. *Oncology Nursing Forum,* 11(6), 46–50.	Perceptions of nurse caring behaviors	Q-sort 50 cards into 7 piles/7 point scale to prioritize perceptions of nurse caring behaviors Noted to be confusing, ambiguous to administer, and time-consuming; but most commonly used, both nationally and internationally	Patients (oncology) n = 57	Expert panel test-retest Content and face validity	General references to nursing theories of caring A priori development Guided by care needs of cancer patients	Chinese version of Care-Q 1998 Holroyd, E., Yue-kuen, C., Sau-wai, C., Fungshan, L., 7 Wai-wan, W. (1998) A Chinese cultural perspective of nursing care behaviors in an acute setting. *Journal of Advanced Nursing,* 28(6), 1289–1294.

TABLE 4.2 (*continued*)

Instrument	Author Contact Address	Publication Citation Source	Developed to Measure	Instrument Description	Participants	Reported Validity/ Reliability	Conceptual/ Theoretical Basis of Measurement	Latest Citation in Nursing Literature
								Hulela, E. B., Akinsola, H. A. & Sekoni, N. M. (2000). The observed nurses caring behavior in a referral hospital in Botswana. *West African Journal of Nursing, 11*(1), 1–6.

(*continued*)

TABLE 4.2 (*continued*)

Instrument	Author Contact Address	Publication Citation Source	Developed to Measure	Instrument Description	Participants	Reported Validity/ Reliability	Conceptual/ Theoretical Basis of Measurement	Latest Citation in Nursing Literature
CARE-Q	Larson, P. (UCSF)	Larson, P. (1986). Cancer nurses' perceptions of caring. *Cancer Nursing*, 9(2), 86–91.	Perceptions of nurse caring behaviors	Q-Sort	Nurses (oncology) n = 57	Extension of Larson, 1984 See Larson, 1984	ditto	ditto

TABLE 4.2 (*continued*)

Instrument	Author Contact Address	Publication Citation Source	Developed to Measure	Instrument Description	Participants	Reported Validity/ Reliability	Conceptual/ Theoretical Basis of Measurement	Latest Citation in Nursing Literature
CARE-Q	Larson, P. (UCSF)	Larson, P. (1987). Comparison of cancer patients and professional nurses' perceptions of important nurse caring behaviors. *Heart & Lung, 16*(2), 187–192.	Identifies nurse caring behaviors	Q-Sort	Nurses (oncology) n = 57 Patients (oncology) n = 57	See Larson, 1984	ditto	ditto

(continued)

33

TABLE 4.2 *(continued)*

Instrument	Author Contact Address	Publication Citation Source	Developed to Measure	Instrument Description	Participants	Reported Validity/ Reliability	Conceptual/ Theoretical Basis of Measurement	Latest Citation in Nursing Literature
CARE-Q Replication study and use	Mayer, D. RN, PhD, Clinical specialist, Mass. General Hospital	Mayer (1987). Oncology nurses vs. cancer patients' perceptions of nurse caring behaviors: A replication study. *Oncology Nursing Forum, 14*(3), 48–52.	Evaluates nurse caring behaviors	Q-Sort	Nurses (oncology) n = 28 Patients (oncology) n = 54	Content and face validity Test-retest reliability (refers to Larson, 1984 original testing)	Replication of instrument; plus extension of conceptual foundation of original Larson (1984) version of Care-Q.	ditto

TABLE 4.2 *(continued)*

Instrument	Author Contact Address	Publication Citation Source	Developed to Measure	Instrument Description	Participants	Reported Validity/ Reliability	Conceptual/ Theoretical Basis of Measurement	Latest Citation in Nursing Literature
CARE-Q	Nori Komorita, PhD, RN Kathleen Doehring, MS, RN Phyllis Hirchert, MS, RN Urbana Regional Program, College of Nursing, U. of Illinois, Urbana	Komorita, N., Doehring, K., Hirchert, P. (1991). Perceptions of caring by nurse educators. *Journal of Nursing Education, 30*(1), 23–29.	Nurse educators' perceptions of caring behaviors	Q-Sort	Nurse Educators n = 110	Refers to Larson's original work (1984)	Caring in relation to nursing education No new reliability or validity reported for nursing educational use	ditto

(continued)

35

TABLE 4.2 *(continued)*

Instrument	Author Contact Address	Publication Citation Source	Developed to Measure	Instrument Description	Participants	Reported Validity/ Reliability	Conceptual/ Theoretical Basis of Measurement	Latest Citation in Nursing Literature
CARE-Q	Antonia Mangold MSN, RN Oncology Clinical Staff Nurse Thomas Jefferson University Hospital, Philadelphia	Manford, A. (1991). Senior nursing students' & Professional Nurses' Perceptions of Effective Caring Behaviors: A Comparative Study. *Journal of Nursing Education,* *30*(3), 134–139.	Identifies and compares nursing students and RNs' perception of caring behaviors	Q-Sort	Nursing Students n = 30	See Larson (1984) Original citation for test-retest reliability	Larson's original conceptual basis; plus informed by Watson's 10 carative factors	ditto

TABLE 4.2 *(continued)*

Instrument	Author Contact Address	Publication Citation Source	Developed to Measure	Instrument Description	Participants	Reported Validity/ Reliability	Conceptual/ Theoretical Basis of Measurement	Latest Citation in Nursing Literature
CARE-Q	Louise von Essen MS, Psychology; Per-Olow Sjoden, PhD Center for Caring Sciences, Uppsala University Akademiska Hospital, S-751 85 Uppsala, SWEDEN *Louise-von.essen@ccs.uu.se*	Von Essen & Sjoden (1991a). The importance of nurse caring behaviors as perceived by Swedish hospital patients and nursing staff. *International Journal of Nursing Studies, 28*(3), 267–281.	Perceived caring behaviors by nurses and patients	Q-Sort **(International Swedish Version)**	Oncology, General Surgery Orthodpedic patients n = 81 Nurses n = 105	No reliability or validity reported for Swedish version Refers to information reported by Larson (1981, 1984)	Affective components of care and a caring relationship	Larsson, G. Petersson, V. W., Lampic, C., von Essen, L., Sjoden, P. (1998). Cancer patient and staff rating of the importance of caring behaviors and their relation to patient anxiety and depression. *Journal of Advanced Nursing, 27,* 855–864.

(continued)

TABLE 4.2 *(continued)*

Instrument	Author Contact Address	Publication Citation Source	Developed to Measure	Instrument Description	Participants	Reported Validity/ Reliability	Conceptual/ Theoretical Basis of Measurement	Latest Citation in Nursing Literature
								Widmark-Petersson, V., von Essen, L. & Sjoden, P. (1998). Perceptions of caring: patients and staff's association to CARE-Q behaviours. *Journal of Psychosocial Oncology, 16*(1), 75–96.

TABLE 4.2 *(continued)*

Instrument	Author Contact Address	Publication Citation Source	Developed to Measure	Instrument Description	Participants	Reported Validity/ Reliability	Conceptual/ Theoretical Basis of Measurement	Latest Citation in Nursing Literature
CARE-Q	Louise von Essen & Per-Olow Sjoden, Uppsala University SWEDEN (see above)	von Essen, & Sjoden, P. (1991). Patient & Staff Perceptions of Caring: Review and Replication. *Journal of Advanced Nursing, 16*(11), 1363–1374.	Perceived caring behaviors by nurses and patients (Swedish population)	**International Version** Q-Sort of same items of 7 point scale (Swedish version) Replication of 1991 study Questionnaires with items of Q-Sort	Nurses n = 73 Medical patients n = 86	See von Essen & Sjoden (1991a)		Widmark-Petersson, V. von Essen, L. & Sjoden, P. (2000). Perceptions of caring among patients with cancer and their staff: differences and disagreements. *Cancer Nursing, 23*(1), 32–39.

(continued)

TABLE 4.2 *(continued)*

Instrument	Author Contact Address	Publication Citation Source	Developed to Measure	Instrument Description	Participants	Reported Validity/ Reliability	Conceptual/ Theoretical Basis of Measurement	Latest Citation in Nursing Literature
CARE-Q	Kathryn Rosenthal, MS, RN University of Colorado	Rosenthal, K. (1992). Coronary care patients' and nurses' perceptions of important nurse caring behaviors. *Heart & Lung, 21*(6), 536–539.	Examines the relationship of patient-perceived and nurse-perceived caring behaviors	Q-Sort	Coronary nurses n = 30 Coronary Patients n = 30	See Larson (1984, 1987)	General nursing caring literature(Larson, 1984, 1987 for tool) Watson et al. included in background of study	None to date

TABLE 4.2 (*continued*)

Instrument	Author Contact Address	Publication Citation Source	Developed to Measure	Instrument Description	Participants	Reported Validity/ Reliability	Conceptual/ Theoretical Basis of Measurement	Latest Citation in Nursing Literature
CARE-Q	Louise von Essen, Per-Olow Sjoden, Uppsala University, Sweden (see above)	Von Essen, L. & Sjoden, P. (1993). Perceived importance of caring behaviors to Swedish psychiatric inpatients and staff with comparisons to somatically-ill samples. *Research in Nursing & Health, 16,* 293–303.	Nurse caring behaviors as perceived by psychiatric patients with comparison to somatically-ill patients	Q-Sort comparative study with different patient populations **International Swedish version of tool modified for psychiatric patients** (used free response format)	Mental Health nurses n = 63 (Psychiatric nurses, RNs, and students) Mental health patients n = 61	Discussion of difficulty with Q-Sort Found to be unreliable due to forced distribution Discusses internal consistency using a free response format Content validity addressed	See above Perception of Caring relationship and caring behaviors	Larsson, G., Pettersson, V. W., Lampic, C., von Essen, L., Sjoden, P. (1998). Cancer patient and staff rating of the importance of caring behaviors and their relation to patient anxiety and depression. *Journal of Advanced Nursing, 27,* 855–864.

(*continued*)

TABLE 4.2 *(continued)*

Instrument	Author Contact Address	Publication Citation Source	Developed to Measure	Instrument Description	Participants	Reported Validity/ Reliability	Conceptual/ Theoretical Basis of Measurement	Latest Citation in Nursing Literature
								Widmark-Petersson, V., von Essen, L., & Sjoden, P. (2000). Perceptions of caring among patients with cancer and their staff: differences and disagreements. *Cancer Nursing, 23*(1), 32–39.

TABLE 4.2 *(continued)*

Instrument	Author Contact Address	Publication Citation Source	Developed to Measure	Instrument Description	Participants	Reported Validity/ Reliability	Conceptual/ Theoretical Basis of Measurement	Latest Citation in Nursing Literature
CARE-Q	Margaret K. Smith, RN, MSN Assistant Nurse Manager, Nursing Home Care Unit VA Palo Alto Health Care System, Menlo Park, CA	Smith, M. (1997). Nurses' and patients' perceptions of most important caring behaviors in a long-term care setting. *Geriatric Nursing, 18*(2), 70–73.	Compare rankings of caring behaviors as perceived by patients and nurses	50 items with 6 sub-scales Q-Sort	n = 12 men; 2 women patients; n = 15 RNs from nursing home care unit at Veterans Affairs Medical Center	Reliability or validity not addressed	No theoretical/conceptual model mentioned	ditto

(continued)

TABLE 4.2 *(continued)*

Instrument	Author Contact Address	Publication Citation Source	Developed to Measure	Instrument Description	Participants	Reported Validity/ Reliability	Conceptual/ Theoretical Basis of Measurement	Latest Citation in Nursing Literature
CARE-Q	Greenhalgh, J., Vanhanen, L., & Kyngas, H. 4 Hayfield Close, Glenfield, Leicester	Greenhalgh, J., Vanhanen, L. & Kyngas, H. (1998). Nurse caring behaviors. *Journal of Advanced Nursing, 27*, 927–932.	Caring behaviors and how they related to nurses practice in psychiatric and general nurses' views	CARE-Q questionnaire with free-choice format **(International use of tool: Finland)**	n = 69 nurses from psychiatric hospital in Northern Finland; n = 49 nurses from general hospital, Northern Finland	Larson (1984)	Caring behaviors from Larson (1984)	

TABLE 4.2 *(continued)*

Instrument	Author Contact Address	Publication Citation Source	Developed to Measure	Instrument Description	Participants	Reported Validity/ Reliability	Conceptual/ Theoretical Basis of Measurement	Latest Citation in Nursing Literature
CARE-Q	Holroyd, E., Yue-kuen, C., Sau-wai, C., Fung-shan, L., & Wai-wan, W. Department of Nursing The Chinese University of Hong Kong	Holroyd, E., Yue-kuen, C., Sau-wai, C., Fung-shan, L. & Wai-wan, W. (1998). *Journal of Advanced Nursing, 28*(6), 1289–1294.	Nursing caring behaviors in an acute care setting	**International Chinese version of CARE-Q** with five-point Likert-type fixed rating measure	n = 29 inpatients from acute public hospital in Hong Kong	Face and content validity based upon Larson (1984) Reliability in test-retest study-item ranking consistency for top 5 items No Chinese version reliability or validity tested	Nurse caring behaviors; Larson (1984)	

(continued)

TABLE 4.2 (*continued*)

Instrument	Author Contact Address	Publication Citation Source	Developed to Measure	Instrument Description	Participants	Reported Validity/ Reliability	Conceptual/ Theoretical Basis of Measurement	Latest Citation in Nursing Literature
CARE-Q (Caring Assessment Instrument)	Larsson, G., Peterson, V. W., Lampic, C., von Essen, L., Sjoden, P. Centre for Caring Sciences, Uppsals University, SWEDEN *Louise-von.essen@ ccs.uu.se*	Larsson, G., Peterson, V. W., Lampic, C., von Essen, L., Sjoden, P. (1998). Cancer patient and staff ratings of the importance of caring behaviors and their relation to patient anxiety and depression. *Journal of Advanced Nursing, 27,* 855–864.	Caring behaviors and patient levels of anxiety and depression in cancer patients	CARE-Q **International version (Swedish)** Larson (1984) von Essen et al. (1994)	n = 53 patients with cancer diagnosis n = 62 staff from 3 units Swedish hospital in Uppsala	Refers to reliability/ validity von Essen & Sjoden (1993)	Caring behaviors original Larson (1994)	**This citation (1998) latest publication of Swedish version of CARE-Q research**

TABLE 4.2 *(continued)*

Instrument	Author Contact Address	Publication Citation Source	Developed to Measure	Instrument Description	Participants	Reported Validity/ Reliability	Conceptual/ Theoretical Basis of Measurement	Latest Citation in Nursing Literature
CARE/ SATISFAC- TION Question- naire (CARE/ SAT) (1993) RE- VISION OF CARE-Q	Patricia Lar- son, DNS, RN(UCSF) Sandra Fer- ketich, PhD, RN Dean, U. of New Mexico	Larson, P. & Ferketich, S. (1993). Pa- tients' satis- faction with nurses' car- ing during hospitaliza- tion. *Western Journal of Nursing Re- search, 15*(6), 690–707.	Patient satis- faction of nursing care	Descriptive correlational study Visual Ana- log scale adapted from CARE-Q; 29 items	n = 268 pa- tients	Cronbach's alpha Construct and concur- rent validity reported Factor analy- sis = 3 factors to account for variance	Original work of Lar- son, with adaptation	

CARE-Q AND CARE/SAT*

DIRECTIONS

THE NURSE CARING BEHAVIOR STUDY

To participate in the study you will be required to sort cards containing statements about nurse caring behaviors, ranking them from most important to least important. See the enclosed directions for the specific details. This will require about 45 to 60 minutes of your time. When you have completed this first phase of the study and mailed it to me (no postage is required) within 30 days I will mail a second CARE-Q (the retest) and have you do the sort again. Individual responses will be kept confidential and every effort will be made to protect your anonymity. Your participation indicates your consent.

> *The purpose of the Nurse Caring Behavior Study is to identify the nurse caring behaviors that are perceived as important in making patients feel cared for.*

The Caring Assessment Report Evaluation Q-Sort (CARE-Q) packet contains seven pockets, each labeled with a number (1, 4, 10, 20, 10, 4, 1). Included in the packet are a deck of 50 cards, each with a different caring nurse behavior typed on it.

To identify the nurse caring behaviors which are perceived as most important, sort the deck of 50 cards from most important to least important, placing each card into one of the pockets—on a range of most important to least important.

It is essential that only the designated number of cards be placed in each pocket, with the numbers (1, 4, 10, 20, etc.) on the pocket indicating the number of cards which can be placed in each pocket. When you have completed the sorting, please count the number of cards in each pocket to make sure that the right number of cards are in each pocket.

Please answer the questions on the Nurse Demographic Information Sheet.

When you have completed the study, place the seven pockets containing the sorted cards and the Nurse Demographic Sheet into the enclosed envelope and mail. No postage is required.

Thank you so much for your help.

(Below is an example of how to place the pockets to aid in the sorting. They are placed from your left to your right).

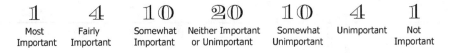

1	4	10	20	10	4	1
Most Important	Fairly Important	Somewhat Important	Neither Important or Unimportant	Somewhat Unimportant	Unimportant	Not Important

---

*©Dr. Patricia Larson. Reprinted with permission of author.

3″ x 5″ cards

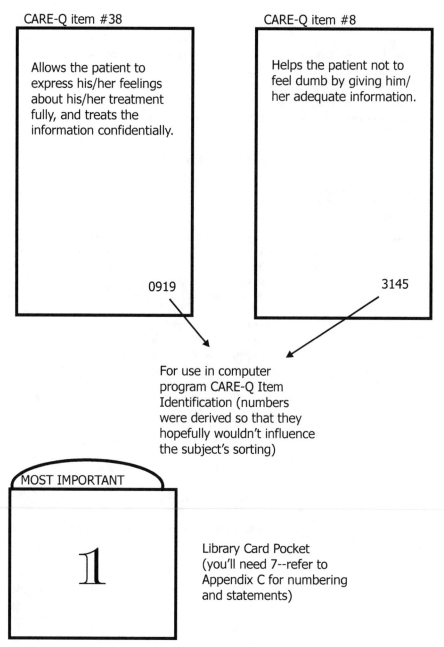

CARE-Q item #38

Allows the patient to express his/her feelings about his/her treatment fully, and treats the information confidentially.

0919

CARE-Q item #8

Helps the patient not to feel dumb by giving him/her adequate information.

3145

For use in computer program CARE-Q Item Identification (numbers were derived so that they hopefully wouldn't influence the subject's sorting)

MOST IMPORTANT

1

Library Card Pocket (you'll need 7--refer to Appendix C for numbering and statements)

CARE-Q

Patients are instructed to sort 50 behaviors according to how important they perceive them to be according to the following question: "In order to make you feel cared for, how important is it that the staff . . . ?" Staff are asked the corresponding question of how important they think each item is in order to make the patient/patients feel cared for. The behaviors are to be ranked in 7 categories from most to least important (1 most and 1 least important item, 4 next most and 4 next least important, 10 rather and 10 not so important, and 20 that are neither important nor unimportant).

ENGLISH VERSION

CARE-Q Items and Scales

Subscales	Item
Accessible	1. Frequently approaches the patient first, e.g., offering such things as pain medication, back rub, etc.
	2. Volunteers to do "little" things for the patient, e.g., brings a cup of coffee, paper, etc.
	3. Gives the patient's treatments and medications on time.
	4. Checks on the patient frequently.
	5. Gives a quick response to the patient's call.
	6. Encourages the patient to call if he/she has problems.
Explains and facilitates	7. Tells the patient of support systems available, such as self-help groups or patients with similar disease.
	8. Helps the patient not to feel dumb by giving him/her adequate information.
	9. Tells the patient, in understandable language, what is important to know about his/her disease and treatment.
	10. Teaches the patient how to care for himself/herself whenever possible.
	11. Suggests questions for the patient to ask her/his doctor.
	12. Is honest with the patient about his medical condition.
Comforts	13. Provides basic comfort measures, such as appropriate lighting, control of noise, adequate blankets, etc.
	14. Provides the patient encouragement by identifying positive elements related to the patient's condition and treatment.
	15. Is patient even with "difficult" patients.
	16. Is cheerful.
	17. Sits down with the patient.

18. Touches the patient when he/she needs comforting.
19. Listens to the patient.
20. Talks to the patient.
21. Involves the patient's family or significant others in their care.

Anticipates

22. Realizes that the nights are frequently the most difficult time for the patient.
23. Anticipates the patient's and her/his family's shock over her/his diagnosis and plans opportunities for them, individually or as a group, to talk about it.
24. Knows when the patient has 'had enough' and acts accordingly, e.g., rearranges an examination, screens visitors, insures privacy.
25. Is perceptive of the patient's needs and plans and acts accordingly, e.g., gives anti-nausea medication when patient is receiving medication which will probably induce nausea.
26. Anticipates that the 'first times' are the hardest and pays special attention to the patient during these times.

Trusting relationship

27. When with a patient, concentrates only on that one patient.
28. Continues to be interested in the patient even though a crisis or critical phase has passed.
29. Offers reasonable alternatives to the patient, such as choice of appointment times, bath times, etc.
30. Helps the patient establish realistic goals.
31. Checks out with the patient the best time to talk with the patient about changes in his/her condition.
32. Checks her/his perceptions of the patient with the patient before initiating any action, e.g., if she/he (the nurse) has the feeling that the patient is upset with the treatment plan, discusses this with the patient before talking about it to the doctor.
33. Helps the patient clarify his thinking in regard to his/her disease and treatments.
34. Realizes that the patient knows himself the best and whenever possible includes the patient in planning and management of his/her care.
35. Encourages the patient to ask her/him any questions he/she might have.
36. Puts the patient first, no matter what else happens.
37. Is pleasant and friendly to the patient's family and significant others.
38. Allows the patient to express his feelings about his/her disease and treatment fully, and treats the information confidentially.
39. Asks the patient what name he/she prefers to be called.

40. Has a consistent approach with the patient.
41. Gets to know the patient as an individual person.
42. Introduces himself/herself and tells the patient what she/he does.

Monitors and follows through

43. Is professional in appearance—wears appropriate identifiable clothing and identification.
44. Makes sure that professional appointment scheduling, e.g., x-ray, special procedures, etc., are realistic to the patient's condition and situation.
45. Is well organized.
46. Knows how to give shots, I.V.s, etc., and how to manage the equipment like I.V.s, suction machines, etc.
47. Is calm.
48. Gives good physical care to the patient.
49. Makes sure others know how to care for the patient
50. Knows when to call the doctor.

SWEDISH VERSION*

CARE-Q beteenden och dimensioner

Dimensioner	Beteenden
Tillgänglighet	1. Tar ofta initiativ till kontakt med patienten, t ex för att ge smärtstillande, massage etc
	2. Erbjuder sig att göra små "ärenden" till patienten, tex att komma med en kopp kaffe, en tidning etc
	3. Ger patienten behandling och mediciner på utlovad tid
	4. Kontrollerar ofta patientens tillstånd
	5. Kommer snabbt då patienten ringer
	6. Uppmuntrar patienten att säga till om han/hon har problem
Förklarar och underlättar	7. Berättar för patienten om var han/hon kan få stöd och hjälp t ex i patientföreningar eller samtalsgrupper
	8. Hjälper patienten att inte känna sig bortkommen genom att ge honom/henne rätt information
	9. Berättar på ett förståeligt språk för patienten det som är viktigt att känna till om sjukdomen och behandlingen
	10. Lär patienten hur han/hon skall ta hand om sig själv då detta är möjligt
	11. Föreslår frågor som patienten kan ställa till sin läkare

*Reprinted with permission of authors.

12. Är uppriktig mot patienten om hans/hennes medicinska tillstånd

Hjälp och tröst

13. Ger patienten hjälp med grundläggande saker som belysning, störande ljud, tillräckligt med sängkläder
14. Ger patienten uppmuntran genom att påpeka positiva inslag i hans/hennes tillstånd och behandling
15. Har tålamod med patienten även om han/hon skulle vara besvärlig
16. Är glad och trevlig
17. Sätter sig ner hos patienten
18. Tar i eller håller om patienten när han/hon behöver tröst
19. Lyssnar på patienten
20. Pratar med patienten
21. Engagerar patientens familj eller andra närstående i vården av honom/henne

Förutseende
uppträdande

22. Inser att natten ofta är den svåraste tidpunkten för patienten
23. Förutser patientens och dennes familjs reaktion på diagnosbeskedet och planerar tillfällen för dem att prata om detta ensamma eller tillsammans
24. Vet när patienten inte "orkar mer" och tar hänsyn till detta, t ex vid undersökningar, ronder, och besök
25. Är uppmärksam på patientens behov och planerar och handlar med tanke på dessa tex genom att ge medel mot illamående om patienten får behandling som brukar framkalla illamående
26. Förutser att första gången en behandling eller en undersökning görs är svårast och ger patienten speciell uppmärksamhet då

Förtroendefullt
uppträdande

27. Koncentrerar sig bara på den patient hon/han är hos och tar en patient i taget
28. Fortsätter att visa intresse för patienten även sedan en kris eller ett kritiskt skede har passerat om patienten skulle få ett sådant
29. Erbjuder patienten rimliga alternativ, t ex när det gäller tider för besök, badtider etc.
30. Hjälper patienten att sätta upp realistiska mål
31. Hör efter med patienten när de bästa tillfällena är att prata om förändringar i hans/hennes tillstånd
32. Kontrollerar sina intryck med patienten innan några åtgärder genomförs, t ex om hon/han uppfattar att patienten är orolig över behandlingsplanen diskuterar honden med patienten innan hon talar med läkaren

33. Hjälper patienten att reda ut sina funderingar kring sjukdomen och behandlingen
34. Inser att patienten känner sig själv bäst, och tar, så ofta det är möjligt, med hans/hennes synpunkter i planering och genomförande av den vård han/hon skall få
35. Uppmuntrar patienten att fråga om saker som han/hon kanske funderar på
36. Sätter patienten främst vad som än händer
37. Är trevlig och vänlig mot patientens familj och andra närstående
38. Tillåter patienten att fritt uttrycka de känslor han/hon har inför sjukdomen och behandlingen, och behandlar denna information konfidentiellt
39. Frågar patienten om vilket namn han/hon vill tilltalas med
40. Är konsekvent i sitt uppträdande mot patienten
41. Lär känna patienten som person
42. Presenterar sig själv och berättar vad hon har för arbetsuppgifter

Professionellt uppträdande

43. Är professionell i sitt uppträdande, har korrekt klädsel och namnskylt
44. Försäkrar sig om att tidsplaneringen för undersökningar och behandling tar hänsyn till patientens situation och tillstånd
45. Har förmågan att organisera sitt arbete
46. Ger injektioner på eft bra sätt, och vet hur man sköter den utrustning som behövs för undersökning och provtagning
47. Är lugn
48. Ger patienten god fysisk vård
49. Försäkrar sig om att andra vet hur patienten skall skötas om
50. Vet när det är dags aft tillkalla läkare

CARING SATISFACTION (CARE/SAT)

THE PURPOSE OF THIS QUESTIONNAIRE IS TO HAVE PATIENTS ASSESS THEIR NURSING CARE. YOUR IMPRESSIONS, ALONG WITH THOSE OF OTHER PATIENTS, WILL HELP NURSES IN DECIDING WAYS TO IMPROVE PATIENT CARE.

EACH STATEMENT REFERS TO A SPECIFIC NURSING ACTION. BASED ON YOUR EXPERIENCE, DECIDE HOW MUCH YOU AGREE OR DISAGREE WITH THE VIEW EXPRESSED. ON THE LINE NEXT TO THE STATEMENT PLACE AN "X" AT THE POINT ALONG THE LINE THAT BEST DESCRIBES HOW MUCH YOU AGREE OR DISAGREE WITH THE STATEMENT. THERE ARE NO RIGHT OR WRONG ANSWERS. YOUR RESPONSE IS A MATTER OF YOUR PERSONAL OPINION. YOUR INDIVIDUAL RESPONSE WILL NOT BE SHARED WITH ANYONE. ONLY GROUP DATA WILL BE REPORTED.

BELOW ARE EXAMPLES WHICH MAY HELP YOU IN RESPONDING TO THE QUESTIONNAIRE.

A. DURING MY HOSPITAL STAY THE NURSES ON THE UNIT:

TAUGHT ME HOW TO   X
TAKE MY TEMPERATURE. _____

                  STRONGLY   STRONGLY
                  DISAGREE   AGREE

THE PLACEMENT OF THE "X" ON THE LINE FOR QUESTION A INDI-CATES THAT YOU DISAGREE BUT NOT TOTALLY, THAT THE NURSES TAUGHT YOU HOW TO TAKE YOUR TEMPERATURE.

B. DURING MY HOSPITAL STAY THE NURSES ON THE UNIT:

DID NOT GIVE MY   X
BATH ON TIME. _____

                  STRONGLY   STRONGLY
                  DISAGREE   AGREE

THE PLACEMENT OF THE "X" FOR QUESTION B IS AN EXAMPLE OF WHERE YOU CANNOT QUITE DECIDE IF YOU AGREE OR DISAGREE BECAUSE AT TIMES YOUR BATH WAS ON TIME AND AT OTHER TIMES IT WAS NOT.

---

*©Patricia J. Larson, R.N., D.N.Sc., Department of Physiological Nursing (N611Y), University of California, San Francisco, San Francisco, California 94114. Telephone (415) 476-1942.

PLACE AN "X" AT THE POINT ON THE LINE THAT BEST DESCRIBES HOW MUCH YOU AGREE OR DISAGREE WITH EACH STATEMENT.

DURING THE PAST WEEK THE NURSES:

1. TOLD ME OF SUP-
PORT SYSTEMS AVAIL-
ABLE TO ME, SUCH
AS SELF-HELP
GROUPS.

_____

STRONGLY   STRONGLY
DISAGREE   AGREE

2. PROVIDED BASIC
COMFORT MEA-
SURES, SUCH AS
APPROPRIATE LIGHT-
ING, CONTROL OF
NOISE, BLANKETS,
ETC.

_____

STRONGLY   STRONGLY
DISAGREE   AGREE

3. ENCOURAGED ME
TO CALL IF I HAD
ANY PROBLEMS.

_____

STRONGLY   STRONGLY
DISAGREE   AGREE

4. DID NOT GIVE A
QUICK RESPONSE TO
MY CALL.

_____

STRONGLY   STRONGLY
DISAGREE   AGREE

5. MADE ME FEEL
DUMB BY GIVING ME
INADEQUATE
INFORMATION.

_____

STRONGLY   STRONGLY
DISAGREE   AGREE

6. DID NOT WANT TO
   TALK ABOUT MY
   FEELINGS ABOUT MY
   DISEASE AND
   TREATMENT.

——————————————————————————————

STRONGLY   STRONGLY
DISAGREE   AGREE

7. APPEARED BUSY AND
   UPSET.

——————————————————————————————

STRONGLY   STRONGLY
DISAGREE   AGREE

8. KNEW WHEN TO
   CALL THE DOCTOR.

——————————————————————————————

STRONGLY   STRONGLY
DISAGREE   AGREE

9. CREATED A SENSE
   OF TRUST FOR ME
   AND MY FAMILY.

——————————————————————————————

STRONGLY   STRONGLY
DISAGREE   AGREE

10. PROVIDED ME EN-
    COURAGEMENT BY
    IDENTIFYING THE
    POSITIVE ASPECTS
    RELATED TO MY
    CONDITION AND
    TREATMENT.

——————————————————————————————

STRONGLY   STRONGLY
DISAGREE   AGREE

11. DID NOT TEACH ME
    HOW TO CARE FOR
    MYSELF.

——————————————————————————————

STRONGLY   STRONGLY
DISAGREE   AGREE

12. ANTICIPATED MY FAMILY'S AND MY SHOCK OVER MY DIAGNOSIS AND PLANNED OPPORTUNITIES, INDIVIDUALLY OR AS A GROUP, TO TALK ABOUT IT.

STRONGLY DISAGREE   STRONGLY AGREE

13. PUT ME FIRST, NO MATTER WHAT ELSE HAPPENED.

STRONGLY DISAGREE   STRONGLY AGREE

14. DID NOT MAKE SURE OTHERS KNEW HOW TO CARE FOR ME.

STRONGLY DISAGREE   STRONGLY AGREE

15. GAVE ME GOOD PHYSICAL CARE.

STRONGLY DISAGREE   STRONGLY AGREE

16. DID NOT HELP ME FIGURE OUT QUESTIONS FOR ME TO ASK MY DOCTOR.

STRONGLY DISAGREE   STRONGLY AGREE

17. VOLUNTEERED TO DO "LITTLE" THINGS SUCH AS BRINGING ME A CUP OF COFFEE, PAPER, ETC.

STRONGLY DISAGREE   STRONGLY AGREE

18. DID *NOT* KNOW MY
    NEEDS WITHOUT
    ME HAVING TO ASK.

    _____
    STRONGLY   STRONGLY
    DISAGREE   AGREE

19. EXPLAINED THINGS
    IMPORTANT TO MY
    CARE.

    _____
    STRONGLY   STRONGLY
    DISAGREE   AGREE

20. CHECKED ON ME
    FREQUENTLY.

    _____
    STRONGLY   STRONGLY
    DISAGREE   AGREE

21. DID NOT GIVE MY
    MEDICATIONS OR
    TREATMENTS ON
    TIME.

    _____
    STRONGLY   STRONGLY
    DISAGREE   AGREE

22. ENCOURAGED ME
    TO ASK ANY QUES-
    TIONS I MIGHT
    HAVE.

    _____
    STRONGLY   STRONGLY
    DISAGREE   AGREE

23. WERE PROFES-
    SIONAL IN
    APPEARANCE.

    _____
    STRONGLY   STRONGLY
    DISAGREE   AGREE

24. KNEW HOW TO
    GIVE SHOTS, I.V.s,
    ETC., AND HOW TO
    MANAGE THE
    EQUIPMENT LIKE
    THE I.V.s, SUCTION
    MACHINES.

    _____
    STRONGLY   STRONGLY
    DISAGREE   AGREE

25. WERE
    DISORGANIZED.

    _____

    STRONGLY   STRONGLY
    DISAGREE   AGREE

26. WERE INCONSIS-
    TENT IN HOW THEY
    TREATED ME.

    _____

    STRONGLY   STRONGLY
    DISAGREE   AGREE

27. DID NOT SEEM TO
    KNOW ME AS A
    PERSON.

    _____

    STRONGLY   STRONGLY
    DISAGREE   AGREE

28. CHECKED WITH ME
    AS TO THE BEST
    TIME TO TALK
    ABOUT CHANCES IN
    MY CONDITION.

    _____

    STRONGLY   STRONGLY
    DISAGREE   AGREE

29. HELPED ME TO
    CLARIFY MY THINK-
    ING IN REGARD TO
    MY DISEASE AND
    TREATMENTS.

    _____

    STRONGLY   STRONGLY
    DISAGREE   AGREE

5

Caring Behaviors Inventory

(Wolf, 1986, 1994)

The Caring Behaviors Inventory (CBI) scale, developed by Wolf (1986, 1994) was the second empirical measurement tool of caring to be reported in the nursing literature (following Larson's publication of the CARE-Q). The conceptual theoretical basis was derived from caring literature in general, and Watson's (1988) Transpersonal Caring Theory, in particular. The conceptual definition reported nurses caring as an "interactive and inter-subjective process that occurs during moments of shared vulnerability between nurse and patient, and that is both both- and other-directed" (Wolf et al., 1994; Beck, 1999).

The CBI is a Likert scale for total scores ranging from 42 to 168. Subjects are asked to rate caring words and phrases on a 4-point scale: 1 = strongly disagree; 2 = disagree; 3 = agree; 4 = strongly agree. This instrument was originally developed with 75 items, and was later revised through psychometric processes, resulting in 42 final items (Wolf et al., 1994; Kyle, 1995; Beck, 1999). There are five correlated subscales within the 42 items: Respectful deference to the other; assurance of human presence; positive connectedness; professional knowledge and skill; attentiveness to the other's experience. Each of these five subscales has a Cronbach's alpha range of .81 (attentiveness to the other's experience) to .92 (assurance of human presence).

The final 42 items were then tested on 541 subjects: 278 nursing staff and 263 patients; the internal consistency reliability was reported to be 0.96 (Wolf, 1994). The highest ranked caring behavior phrase was identified as "attentive listening," comparable with findings in the studies using the CARE-Q instrument (Kyle, 1995). After the 1994 study, the Likert scale of the CBI was revised to increase the variability of responses, increasing the scale from a 4-point to a 6-point Likert, with 1 = never; 4 = usually; 5 = almost always; 6 = always. Additional studies have slightly altered the directions for the instrument to conform to investigators needs with different populations of either nurses or patients.

Additional reports of the instrument use and refinements are found in the following publications: Wolf, Z. R., Colahan, M., Costello, A., Warwick, F., Ambrose, M. S., & Giardino, E. R. (1998). Relationship between nurse caring and patient satisfaction. *MEDSURG Nursing, 7*(2), 99–105. In this study the reading level was 5.9 and reading ease was 60.7 (Flesch-Kincaid); the overall Cronbach's alpha coefficient was 0.98. A study by Swan (1998) reported a .96 alpha with a patient population of 100.

The CBI is considered to be a second-generation instrument in measuring caring. It is one of the earliest to be developed with clarity of conceptual-theoretical basis, along with on-going testing and refinement of instrument. It is one of the few instruments in caring that provides supportive evidence for empirical validation of Watson's Transpersonal Caring Theory. This is a promising tool, having been reported to be among those with the shortest length of time to complete (ranking second, among a set of five caring instruments) taking 12.38 minutes; it has been noted to have consistent language, with easy to understand instructions, and easy to analyze results, which could be used in a correlational design study; it has been described as being valuable in determining perceptions of caring in both patients and nurses (Andrews, Daniels, & Hall, 1996). The author retains copyright of the instrument and requests that anyone wishing to use contact her for both permission, further advice, and follow-up testing. A matrix of the CBI follows in Table 5.1.

TABLE 5.1 Matrix of Caring Behavior Inventory (Wolf, 1986)

Instrument and Year Developed	Author Contact Address	Year Published Source Citation	Developed to Measure	Instrument Description	Participants	Reported Reliability/ Validity	Conceptual-Theoretical Basis	Latest Citation to Date
Caring Behavior Inventory (CBI) 1981, 1983, 1986	Zane Wolf, RN, PhD, La Salle University School of Nursing, 1900 West Olney Ave. Philadelphia, PA 19141 *wolf@lasalle.edu* Ph: (215) 951-1432 Fax: (215) 951-1896	Wolf, Z. R. (1986). The caring concept & nurse identified caring behaviors. *Topics in Clinical Nursing,* 8(2), 84–93.	Words, phrases in nursing literature that represent caring (attitudes and actions)	42 final items, derived from 75 original words/phrases 4-point Likert Scale; easy to use; brief to administer	Nurses n = 97	Content validity from literature sources	Strongly informed by Watson theory (1988); refers to transpersonal and 10 carative factors	Wolf et al. (1998). Research Utilization: Relationship between nurse caring and patient satisfaction. *MEDSURG Nursing,* 7(2), 99–105.

(continued)

TABLE 5.1 *(continued)*

Instrument and Year Developed	Author Contact Address	Year Published Source Citation	Developed to Measure	Instrument Description	Participants	Reported Reliability/ Validity	Conceptual-Theoretical Basis	Latest Citation to Date
								Swan, B. A. (1998). Research utilization. Postoperative nursing care contributions to symptom distress and functional status after ambulatory surgery. *Medsurg. Nursing,* 7(3), 148–151.

TABLE 5.1 *(continued)*

Instrument and Year Developed	Author Contact Address	Year Published Source Citation	Developed to Measure	Instrument Description	Participants	Reported Reliability/ Validity	Conceptual- Theoretical Basis	Latest Citation to Date
CBI revised 1986, 1994	Zane Wolf (above)	Wolf, Z., et al. (1994). Dimensions of nurse caring. *Image: Journal of Nursing Scholarship, 26*(2), 107–111.	Process of caring	4-point Likert (suggested to use 7-point Likert) 42-items based on words/phrases	Nurses n = 278 Patients n = 263	Test-retest reliability 0.96 on 278 nurses; content & construct validity— expert panel; factor analysis: 5 items; 42 items	Watson's theory; transpersonal dimensions	See Wolf et al. (1998)

(continued)

TABLE 5.1 *(continued)*

Instrument and Year Developed	Author Contact Address	Year Published Source Citation	Developed to Measure	Instrument Description	Participants	Reported Reliability/ Validity	Conceptual-Theoretical Basis	Latest Citation to Date
CBI 1998 Retesting	Dr. Zane Wolf See above	Wolf et al. (1998). Relationship between nurse caring and patient satisfaction. *MEDSURG Nursing,* 7(2), 99–105.	Retesting with adult patients caring process and actions	Original instrument with 6-point Likert scale	n = 335 Adult hospitalized medical surgical patients	Overall Cronbach's alpha 0.98; reading level reported at 5.9 and reading ease at 60.7.	Watson's Transpersonal Caring Theory	Wolf et al. (1998). Relationship between nurse caring and patient satisfaction. *MEDSURG Nursing,* 7(2), 99–105.

CARING BEHAVIORS INVENTORY I
(Wolf, 1988)

Directions:

Nurses do many things when they care for patients. Below is a list of responses that may represent nurse caring. Please read each phrase and indicate if you agree or disagree that the phrase indicates nurse caring.

Kindly use the scale provided to select your answer. Please circle the number you select after reading each item.

1 = strongly disagree
2 = disagree
3 = agree
4 = strongly agree

1.	Attentively listening to the patient.	1	2	3	4
2.	Giving instructions or teaching the patient.	1	2	3	4
3.	Treating the patient as an individual.	1	2	3	4
4.	Spending time with the patient.	1	2	3	4
5.	Touching the patient to communicate caring.	1	2	3	4
6.	Being hopeful for the patient.	1	2	3	4
7.	Giving the patient information so that he or she can make a decision.	1	2	3	4
8.	Showing respect for the patient.	1	2	3	4
9.	Supporting the patient.	1	2	3	4
10.	Calling the patient by his/her preferred name.	1	2	3	4
11.	Being honest with the patient.	1	2	3	4
12.	Trusting the patient.	1	2	3	4
13.	Being empathetic or identifying with the patient.	1	2	3	4
14.	Helping the patient grow.	1	2	3	4
15.	Making the patient physically or emotionally comfortable.	1	2	3	4
16.	Being sensitive to the patient.	1	2	3	4
17.	Being patient or tireless with the patient.	1	2	3	4
18.	Helping the patient.	1	2	3	4
19.	Knowing how to give shots, IVs, etc.	1	2	3	4

---

*©Zane Robinson Wolf, PhD, RN, FAAN. Reprinted with permission of author.

20.	Being confident with the patient.	1	2	3	4
21.	Using a soft, gentle voice with the patient.	1	2	3	4
22.	Demonstrating professional knowledge and skill.	1	2	3	4
23.	Watching over the patient.	1	2	3	4
24.	Managing equipment skillfully.	1	2	3	4
25.	Being cheerful with the patient.	1	2	3	4
26.	Allowing the patient to express feelings about his or her disease and treatment.	1	2	3	4
27.	Including the patient in planning his or her care.	1	2	3	4
28.	Treating patient information confidentially.	1	2	3	4
29.	Providing a reassuring presence.	1	2	3	4
30.	Returning to the patient voluntarily.	1	2	3	4
31.	Talking with the patient.	1	2	3	4
32.	Encouraging the patient to call if there are problems.	1	2	3	4
33.	Meeting the patient's stated and unstated needs.	1	2	3	4
34.	Responding quickly to the patient's call.	1	2	3	4
35.	Appreciating the patient as a human being.	1	2	3	4
36.	Helping to reduce the patient' s pain.	1	2	3	4
37.	Showing concern for the patient.	1	2	3	4
38.	Giving the patient's treatments and medications on time.	1	2	3	4
39.	Paying special attention to the patient during first times, as hospitalization, treatments.	1	2	3	4
40.	Relieving the patient's symptoms.	1	2	3	4
41.	Putting the patient first.	1	2	3	4
42.	Giving good physical care.	1	2	3	4

Please complete the following information:

Patient Profile:

Patients are asked to complete this section.

1. Sex: 1. female   2. male

2. Age: _____

3. Marital Status:
    1. single
    2. married
    3. divorced
    4. widowed
    5. separated

4. Race
    1. African American _____
    2. Asian _____
    3. Caucasian _____
    4. Hispanic _____
    5. Native American Indian _____
    6. Other, please specify _____

5. Educational Level:
    1. 1–8 grade _____
    2. 9–12 grade _____
    3. 1–2 years college _____
    4. 3–4 years college _____
    5. 5 years college and over _____

6. Highest degree earned _____

7. Type of health care setting where you were cared for by nurses:
    1. university hospital _____
    2. suburban/community hospital hospital _____
    3. long term care facility _____
    4. nursing home _____
    5. community health nursing agency _____
    6. senior citizen center _____
    7. other, please specify _____

8. Number of admissions to hospital or other health care setting in the last 5 years _____

9.   Reason for last admission or need for health care services of nurse

_____

10.   Number of days in hospital or other health care setting during the
      last admission _____

Nurse Profile:

Nursing staff are asked to complete this section.

1.   Sex: 1. female   2. male

2.   Age: _____

3.   Marital Status:
     1.   single
     2.   married
     3.   divorced
     4.   widowed
     5.   separated

4.   Race
     1.   African American _____
     2.   Asian _____
     3.   Caucasian _____
     4.   Hispanic _____
     5.   Native American Indian _____
     6.   Other, please specify _____

5.   Educational Level:
     1.   1–8 grade _____
     2.   9–12 grade _____
     3.   1–2 years college _____
     4.   3–4 years college _____
     5.   5 years college and over _____

6.   Work place (for example, hospital, nursing home, home
     care): _____

7.   Highest degree earned: _____

8.   Position in nursing:
     1.   NA—nursing assistant staff _____
     2.   LPN—staff nurse _____
     3.   RN—staff nurse _____

   4. RN—nurse manager _____
   5. RN—assistant nurse manager _____
   6. RN—supervisor _____
   7. RN—care coordinator _____
   8. RN—director of nursing _____
   9. RN—nursing faculty _____
 10. other, please specify _____

©Zane Robinson Wolf, 1981; 1990; 1991; 10/91; 1/92.

CARING BEHAVIORS INVENTORY II

Directions:
Below is a list of the responses that represent nurse caring. For each item, rank the extent that a nurse or nurses made each response visible.

Please use the scale provided to select your answer. Circle the number you select after reading each item.

1 = never
2 = almost never
3 = occasionally
4 = usually
5 = almost always
6 = always

1.	Attentively listening to the patient.	1	2	3	4	5	6
2.	Giving instructions or teaching the patient.	1	2	3	4	5	6
3.	Treating the patient as an individual.	1	2	3	4	5	6
4.	Spending time with the patient.	1	2	3	4	5	6
5.	Touching the patient to communicate caring.	1	2	3	4	5	6
6.	Being hopeful for the patient.	1	2	3	4	5	6
7.	Giving the patient information so that he or she can make a decision.	1	2	3	4	5	6
8.	Showing respect for the patient.	1	2	3	4	5	6
9.	Supporting the patient.	1	2	3	4	5	6
10.	Calling the patient by his/her preferred name.	1	2	3	4	5	6

11.	Being honest with the patient.	1	2	3	4	5	6
12.	Trusting the patient.	1	2	3	4	5	6
13.	Being empathetic or identifying with the patient.	1	2	3	4	5	6
14.	Helping the patient grow.	1	2	3	4	5	6
15.	Making the patient physically or emotionally comfortable.	1	2	3	4	5	6
16.	Being sensitive to the patient.	1	2	3	4	5	6
17.	Being patient or tireless with the patient.	1	2	3	4	5	6
18.	Helping the patient.	1	2	3	4	5	6
19.	Knowing how to give shots, IVs, etc.	1	2	3	4	5	6
20.	Being confident with the patient.	1	2	3	4	5	6
21.	Using a soft, gentle voice with the patient.	1	2	3	4	5	6
22.	Demonstrating professional knowledge and skill.	1	2	3	4	5	6
23.	Watching over the patient.	1	2	3	4	5	6
24.	Managing equipment skillfully.	1	2	3	4	5	6
25.	Being cheerful with the patient.	1	2	3	4	5	6
26.	Allowing the patient to express feelings about his or her disease and treatment.	1	2	3	4	5	6
27.	Including the patient in planning his or her care.	1	2	3	4	5	6
28.	Treating patient information confidentially.	1	2	3	4	5	6
29.	Providing a reassuring presence.	1	2	3	4	5	6
30.	Returning to the patient voluntarily.	1	2	3	4	5	6
31.	Talking with the patient.	1	2	3	4	5	6
32.	Encouraging the patient to call if there are problems.	1	2	3	4	5	6
33.	Meeting the patient's stated and unstated needs.	1	2	3	4	5	6
34.	Responding quickly to the patient's call.	1	2	3	4	5	6
35.	Appreciating the patient as a human being.	1	2	3	4	5	6
36.	Helping to reduce the patient's pain.	1	2	3	4	5	6

37.	Showing concern for the patient.	1	2	3	4	5	6
38.	Giving the patient's treatments and medications on time.	1	2	3	4	5	6
39.	Paying special attention to the patient during first times, as hospitalization, treatments.	1	2	3	4	5	6
40.	Relieving the patient's symptoms.	1	2	3	4	5	6
41.	Putting the patient first.	1	2	3	4	5	6
42.	Giving good physical care.	1	2	3	4	5	6

Please complete the following information:

Patient Profile:

Patients are asked to complete this section.

1. Sex: 1. female   2. male

2. Age: _____

3. Marital Status:
   1. single
   2. married
   3. divorced
   4. widowed
   5. separated

4. Race
   1. African American _____
   2. Asian _____
   3. Caucasian _____
   4. Hispanic _____
   5. Native American Indian _____
   6. Other, please specify _____

5. Educational Level:
   1. 1–8 grade _____
   2. 9–12 grade _____
   3. 1–2 years college _____
   4. 3–4 years college _____
   5. 5 years college and over _____

6. Highest degree earned _____

7. Type of health care setting where you were cared for by nurses:
    1. university hospital _____
    2. suburban/community hospital hospital _____
    3. long term care facility _____
    4. nursing home _____
    5. community health nursing agency _____
    6. senior citizen center _____
    7. other, please specify _____

8. Number of admissions to hospital or other health care setting in the last 5 years _____

9. Reason for last admission or need for health care services of nurse
    _____

10. Number of days in hospital or other health care setting during the last admission _____

Nurse Profile:

Nursing staff are asked to complete this section.

1. Sex: 1. female   2. male

2. Age: _____

3. Marital Status:
    1. single
    2. married
    3. divorced
    4. widowed
    5. separated

4. Race
    1. African American _____
    2. Asian _____
    3. Caucasian _____
    4. Hispanic _____
    5. Native American Indian _____
    6. Other, please specify _____

5. Educational Level:
    1. 1–8 grade _____
    2. 9–12 grade _____

3. 1–2 years college _____
4. 3–4 years college _____
5. 5 years college and over _____

6. Work place (for example, hospital, nursing home, home care): _____

7. Highest degree earned: _____

8. Position in nursing:
    1. NA—nursing assistant staff _____
    2. LPN—staff nurse _____
    3. RN—staff nurse _____
    4. RN—nurse manager _____
    5. RN—assistant nurse manager _____
    6. RN—supervisor _____
    7. RN—care coordinator _____
    8. RN—director of nursing _____
    9. RN—nursing faculty _____
    10. other, please specify _____

©Zane Robinson Wolf, 1981: 1990; 1991; 10/91; 1/92, 3/92; 8/94.

RELEASE FORM FOR THE CARING BEHAVIORS
INVENTORY (CBI)
(WOLF, 1986, 1994)

Name ———————————— Degrees ————————————

Address ——————————————————————————————

——————————————————————————————

——————————————————————————————

Phone   (work) ——————————————————————————

(home) ——————————————————————————

1. Very briefly describe your research project:

2. Estimate how many subjects will complete the CBI:

3. If the research project involves a thesis or dissertation, give the major advisor's name and address below:

I agree to share the results of my study with Zane Robinson Wolf. They will add the results to their database. I will also give them descriptive information about subjects who completed the CBI.

————————————————————————   ————————————

Signature   Date

Please retain one copy of this form for your records and send the original back in the self-addressed stamped envelope.

Zane Robinson Wolf
wolf@lasalle.edu
La Salle University School of Nursing
1900 West Olney Avenue
Philadelphia, PA 19141
Fax: (215) 951-1896

6

Caring Behaviors Assessment Tool

(Cronin and Harrison, 1988)

The Caring Behaviors Assessment (CBA) tool is one of the early tools developed to assess caring. It was the first one reported in the nursing literature to have an explicit theoretical-conceptual basis from which to derive the specific items. It is based upon Watson's (1985, 1988) theory and the 10 carative factors identified in her work.

The original work was developed by Cronin and Harrison (1988). The CBA consists of 63 nurse caring behaviors that are grouped into 7 subscales that are congruent with Watson's carative factors. The first three of the 10 carative factors are grouped together into one subscale, which is conceptually congruent with Watson's theory. The sixth carative factor, "use of a creative, problem-solving, caring process," was assumed by the authors to be inherent in all aspects of nursing care, making it imperceptible to patients. The tool was developed with language that was written at the sixth-grade level. The items are rated on a 5-point Likert scale, to reflect the degree to which each nursing behavior reflects caring.

The original research was conducted on a sample of 22 coronary patients who had a myocardial infarction. Content validity was assessed by four experts familiar with Watson's caring theory. Cronin and Harrison (1988) took into account readability and reliability, as well as face and content validity. The internal consistency reliabilities originally reported were based on Cronbach's alpha (Cronin & Harrison, 1988) and later assessed by Huggins et al. (1993). They included the following rates on specific subscales (Cronin & Harrison, 1988):

Humanism/faith-hope-sensitivity	0.84
Helping/trust	0.76

Expression of positive/negative	0.67
Teaching/learning	0.90
Supportive/p rotective/corrective	0.79
Human need/assistance	0.89
Existential/phenomenological	0.66

Similar reliability rates were reported by Huggins et al. (1993) with a sample of 288 ambulatory patients accessed in an emergency room. Moreover, the CBA has been used also to measure caring behaviors with 19 surgical patients and 46 adults with AIDS or HIV (Parsons et al., 1993; Mullins, 1996), but these last two studies did not report on reliability (Kyle, 1995; Beck, 1999). However, a later study by Schultz et al. (1999) reported an additional test of reliability, with a range of .71 to .88 for the subscales, and an alpha of .93 for the total scale. The most recent report of the instrument's use is by Manogin, Bechtel, and Rami (2000) with a group of childbearing women. In this study, they report Cronbach's alpha reliability for each of the seven subscales, which ranged from .66 to .90. A panel of experts confirmed face and content validity.

In the original research, the two specific items found to be the most important, as perceived by patients were: "makes me feel someone is there if I need them" and "know what they are doing." The least important items were: "visits me when I move to another hospital unit" and "asks me what I like to be called." These findings have been interpreted to suggest that the most important caring behaviors, as perceived by the patient, were those demonstrating professional competence. However, Cronin and Harrison (1988) caution against jumping to such conclusions, suggesting limitations of the CBA, including length and variability in items listed (Kyle, 1995; Beck, 1999). This instrument is copyrighted by the authors and developers of the CBA, and they request that anyone using the instrument contact them. The following Table 6.1 summarizes the status of the CBA in the form of a matrix.

TABLE 6.1 Matrix of Caring Behavior Assessment Tool (Cronin & Harrison, 1988)

Instrument/ Year Developed	Author Contact Address	Year Published/ Source Citation	Developed to Measure	Instrument Description	Participants	Reported Reliability/ Validity	Theoretical-Conceptual Basis	Latest Citation in Nursing Literature
Caring Behavior Assessment Instrument (CBA) 1988	Sherill Cronin, RN, PhD & Barbara Harrison, MEd., RN, Lansing School of Nursing, Bellarmine Nursing, Bellarmine College, Newburg Road, Louisville, KY 40205-0671 *scronin@ bellarmine. edu*	Cronin, S., & Harrison, B. (1988). Importance of nurse caring behaviors as perceived by patients after myocardial infarction. *Heart and Lung, 17*(4), 374–380.	Patient's perception of nurse caring behaviors; explicitly attempts to address process	63 items 7 subscales 5-point Likert rating	Post-myocardial infarction patients n = 22	Cronbach's alpha established; face and content validity obtained	Watson's Theory of caring and 10 carative factors in theory	Manogin, T. W., Bechtel, G., & Rami, R. (2000). Caring behaviors by nurses: Women's perceptions during childbirth. *JOGNN, 29*(2), 153–157.

(continued)

TABLE 6.1 *(continued)*

Instrument/ Year Developed	Author Contact Address	Year Published/ Source Citation	Developed to Measure	Instrument Description	Participants	Reported Reliability/ Validity	Theoretical-Conceptual Basis	Latest Citation in Nursing Literature
CBA (further testing)	Margaret Helene Stanfield, PhD Texas Women's University	Stanfield, M. H. (1991). *Watson's caring theory and instrument development. Dissertation Abstracts International,* 52(8), 4128–B. Order No. DA 9203096. 158 pp.	Patients' perceptions of caring	63 items 7 subscales, based on Watson's carative factors	N = 104 adult hospitalized patients medical-surgical unit	Alpha for whole instrument .9566; subscales, alpha .7825–.8867; construct validity established with factor analysis	Watson's theory of caring and 10 carative factors	

TABLE 6.1 *(continued)*

Instrument/ Year Developed	Author Contact Address	Year Published/ Source Citation	Developed to Measure	Instrument Description	Participants	Reported Reliability/ Validity	Theoretical-Conceptual Basis	Latest Citation in Nursing Literature
CBA (revised) 1993	Elizabeth Parsons, MSN, RN, Carolyn Kee, PhD, RN, Crawford, W. Long Hospital of Emory University, Atlanta, Georgia	Parson, E., Kee, C., et al. (1993). Perioperative Nursing Caring Behaviors. *AORN Journal, 57*(5), 1106–1114.	Patients' perceptions of nurse caring behaviors	63 items, 5-point Likert, 7 subscales (revised original CBA)	Post surgery patients (short stay) n = 19	Based upon Cronin & Harrison (1988)	Watson caring theory and 10 carative factors	ditto

(continued)

TABLE 6.1 (continued)

Instrument/ Year Developed	Author Contact Address	Year Published/ Source Citation	Developed to Measure	Instrument Description	Participants	Reported Reliability/ Validity	Theoretical- Conceptual Basis	Latest Citation in Nursing Literature
CBA (revised) 1993	Kathleen Huggins, MSN, RN, William Gandy, EdD, & Catherine Kohut Baptist Memorial Hospital, Memphis, TN	Huggins, K., Gandy, W., & Kohut, C. (1993). Emergency department patient perceptions of nurse caring behaviors. *Heart and Lung, 22(4),* L356–364.	Patients' perceptions of nurse caring behaviors	Modified for phone survey & emergency patients 65 items; 4-point ordinal; 6 subscales	Emergency Patients n = 288	Original reports of Cronin & Harrison (1988)	Watson theory/10 carative factors	ditto

TABLE 6.1 *(continued)*

Instrument/ Year Developed	Author Contact Address	Year Published/ Source Citation	Developed to Measure	Instrument Description	Participants	Reported Reliability/ Validity	Theoretical-Conceptual Basis	Latest Citation in Nursing Literature
CBA original	Iris L. Mullins Auburn University, School of Nursing, Auburn, AL	Mullins, I. L. (1996). *Nurse caring behaviors for persons with AIDS/HIV. Applied Nursing Research,* 9(1), 18–23.	Identify caring behaviors desired by patients with AIDS/HIV	63 nurse caring behaviors, open-ended question at end of CBA	n = 46 from AIDS outreach groups and AIDS support groups; 4 geographical areas in SE USA	Reliability and validity from Cronin & Harrison (1988)	Watson theory and carative factors as rationale for selecting CBA	ditto

(continued)

TABLE 6.1 (continued)

Instrument/ Year Developed	Author Contact Address	Year Published/ Source Citation	Developed to Measure	Instrument Description	Participants	Reported Reliability/ Validity	Theoretical- Conceptual Basis	Latest Citation in Nursing Literature
CBA Original Cronin & Harrison version	Schultz, C. Bridgham, M. E., Smith, & D. Higgins: Schultz, RN, PhD, nurse researcher, Maine Medical Center (MMC); Bridgham, RN, BSN Head Nurse Maternity Unit, Maine Medical Center; Mary Smith, RN, BSN, Assistant Head Nurse, Maternity, MMC; Diane Higgins, RN, BSN Staff Nurse MCC	Schultz, A. A., Bridgham, C., Smith, M. E., & Higgins, D. (1998). Perceptions of caring. Comparison of antepartum and postpartum patients. *Clinical Nursing Research,* 7, 363–378.	Describe and compare similarities and differences in the perceptions of caring behaviors between antepartum patients and short-term postpartum patients	CBA as developed by Cronin and Harrison (1988) 63 caring behaviors; 5-point Likert scale	n = 42 convenience sample of antepartum and short-term postpartum patients	Reports additional test of reliability; .71–.88 for subscales; alpha of .93 for total scale	Watson's theory; carative factors	ditto

TABLE 6.1 *(continued)*

Instrument/ Year Developed	Author Contact Address	Year Published/ Source Citation	Developed to Measure	Instrument Description	Participants	Reported Reliability/ Validity	Theoretical- Conceptual Basis	Latest Citation in Nursing Literature
CBA Original	B. Marini, RN, MSN Educator, Continuing Education, Department of Nursing & Allied Health, Bucks County Community College Newtown, PA 705 Darley Circle, New Hope, PA 18938	Marini, B. (1999). Institutionalized older adults' perceptions of nurse caring behaviors. *Journal of Gerontological Nursing, 25*(5), 11–16.	Perceptions of caring from older adults, institutionalized	CBA with 64 nurse caring behaviors, with 7 subscales; plus 1 open-ended question "Is there anything else that nurses do to make you feel cared for or about?"	21 residents in long-term care, assisted-living facility	Additional correlations established on subscales by gender; highest range 0.89 for women; 0.85 for men	Watson's theory; carative factors	ditto

(continued)

TABLE 6.1 *(continued)*

Instrument/ Year Developed	Author Contact Address	Year Published/ Source Citation	Developed to Measure	Instrument Description	Participants	Reported Reliability/ Validity	Theoretical-Conceptual Basis	Latest Citation in Nursing Literature
CBA Original	S. Gay, RN, MSN Staff Nurse; Intensive Care Unit St. Francis Hospital, Beech Grove, Indiana	Gay, S. (1999). Meeting cardiac patients' expectations of caring. *Dimensions of Critical Care Nursing*, 18(4), 46–50.	Importance of caring to cardiac patients	CBA 63 items	$n = 18$ Hospitalized cardiac patients	Report content and face validity with use of panel of experts familiar with Watson's theory; reliability Cronbach's alpha .66–.90.	Watson's caring theory; carative factors	ditto

TABLE 6.1 *(continued)*

Instrument/ Year Developed	Author Contact Address	Year Published/ Source Citation	Developed to Measure	Instrument Description	Participants	Reported Reliability/ Validity	Theoretical- Conceptual Basis	Latest Citation in Nursing Literature
CBA Original	Toni Winfield Manogin, Assistant Professor; Gregory Bechtel, Professor Graduate Programs Nursing; Janet Rami, Dean, School of Nursing, Southern University School of Nursing, 11161 Paddock Avenue, Baton Rouge, LA 70816 *Gbechtel@ earthlink.net.*	Manogin, T. W., Bechtel, G., & Rami, R. (2000). Caring behaviors by nurses: Women's perceptions during childbirth. *JOGNN*, *29*(2), 153–157.	Perception of nurse caring behaviors by women during childbirth	CBA 63 items; 7 subscales	Convenience sample; n = 31 women hospitalized for uncomplicated labor and delivery	Expert panel for content validity; Cronbach's alpha for each of 7 subscales ranged from .66 to .90.	Watson's caring theory and carative factors; earlier work of Cronin & Harrison	ditto

CARING BEHAVIORS ASSESSMENT TOOL*

Listed below are things nurses might do or say to make you feel cared for and about. Please decide how important each of these would be in making you feel cared for and about. For each item, indicate if it would be of:

Much Importance   Little Importance
    5   4   3   2   1

Please circle the number that tells you how important each item would be to you.

1.	Treat me as an individual.	5	4	3	2	1
2.	Try to see things from my point of view.	5	4	3	2	1
3.	Know what they're doing.	5	4	3	2	1
4.	Reassure me.	5	4	3	2	1
5.	Make me feel someone is there if I need them.	5	4	3	2	1
6.	Encourage me to believe in myself.	5	4	3	2	1
7.	Point out positive things about me and my condition.	5	4	3	2	1
8.	Praise my efforts.	5	4	3	2	1
9.	Understand me.	5	4	3	2	1
10.	Ask me how I like things done.	5	4	3	2	1
11.	Accept me the way I am.	5	4	3	2	1
12.	Be sensitive to my feelings and moods.	5	4	3	2	1
13.	Be kind and considerate.	5	4	3	2	1
14.	Know when I've "had enough" and act accordingly (for example, limiting visitors).	5	4	3	2	1
15.	Maintain a calm manner.	5	4	3	2	1
16.	Treat me with respect.	5	4	3	2	1
17.	Really listen to me when I talk.	5	4	3	2	1
18.	Accept my feelings without judging them.	5	4	3	2	1
19.	Come into my room just to check on me.	5	4	3	2	1
20.	Talk to me about my life outside the hospital.	5	4	3	2	1
21.	Ask me what I like to be called.	5	4	3	2	1
22.	Introduce themselves to me.	5	4	3	2	1

---

*Reprinted with permission of authors. Users who wish to reproduce this tool must request permission from authors.
*©Copyright Cronin & Harrison.

23.	Answer quickly when I call for them.	5	4	3	2	1
24.	Give me their full attention when with me.	5	4	3	2	1
25.	Visit me if I move to another hospital unit.	5	4	3	2	1
26.	Touch me when I need it for comfort.	5	4	3	2	1
27.	Do what they say they will do.	5	4	3	2	1
28.	Encourage me to talk about how I feel.	5	4	3	2	1
29.	Don't become upset when I'm angry.	5	4	3	2	1
30.	Help me understand my feelings.	5	4	3	2	1
31.	Don't give up on me when I'm difficult to get along with.	5	4	3	2	1
32.	Encourage me to ask questions about my illness and treatment.	5	4	3	2	1
33.	Answer my questions clearly.	5	4	3	2	1
34.	Teach me about my illness.	5	4	3	2	1
35.	Ask me questions to be sure I understand.	5	4	3	2	1
36.	Ask me what I want to know about my health/illness.	5	4	3	2	1
37.	Help me set realistic goals for my health.	5	4	3	2	1
38.	Help me plan ways to meet those goals.	5	4	3	2	1
39.	Help me plan for my discharge from the hospital.	5	4	3	2	1
40.	Tell me what to expect during the day.	5	4	3	2	1
41.	Understand when I need to be alone.	5	4	3	2	1
42.	Offer things (position changes, blankets, back rub, lighting, etc.) to make me more comfortable.	5	4	3	2	1
43.	Leave my room neat after working with me.	5	4	3	2	1
44.	Explain safety precautions to me and my family.	5	4	3	2	1
45.	Give me pain medication when I need it.	5	4	3	2	1
46.	Encourage me to do what I can for myself.	5	4	3	2	1
47.	Respect my modesty (for example, keeping me covered).	5	4	3	2	1
48.	Check with me before leaving the room to be sure I have everything I need within reach.	5	4	3	2	1
49.	Consider my spiritual needs.	5	4	3	2	1
50.	Are gentle with me.	5	4	3	2	1
51.	Are cheerful.	5	4	3	2	1
52.	Help me with my care until I'm able to do it for myself.	5	4	3	2	1

53.	Know how to give shots, IVs, etc.	5	4	3	2	1
54.	Know how to handle equipment (for example, monitors).	5	4	3	2	1
55.	Give me treatments and medicatIons on time.	5	4	3	2	1
56.	Keep my family informed of my progress.	5	4	3	2	1
57.	Let my family visit as much as possible.	5	4	3	2	1
58.	Check my condition very closely.	5	4	3	2	1
59.	Help me feel like I have some control.	5	4	3	2	1
60.	Know when it's necessary to call the doctor.	5	4	3	2	1
61.	Seem to know how I feel.	5	4	3	2	1
62.	Help me see that my past experiences are important.	5	4	3	2	1
63.	Help me feel good about myself.	5	4	3	2	1

Is there anything else that nurses could do or say to make you feel cared for and about? If so, what?

TITLE: Caring Behaviors Assessment (CBA)
AUTHORS: Sherill Nones Cronin, RN, C, PhD
Barbara Harrison, RN, C, MSN

Development of the CBA

The Caring Behaviors Assessment (CBA) was developed to assess the relative contribution of identified nursing behaviors to the patient's sense of feeling cared for and about.

The original CBA listed 61 nursing behaviors, ordered in seven subscales which are congruent with Watson's carative factors. The subscales, with their respective item numbers and corresponding reliabilities, are:

Subscale	Items	Cronbach alpha
Humanism/faith-hope/ sensitivity	1–16	.84
Helping/trust	17–27	.76
Expression of positive/ negative feelings	28–31	.67
Teaching/learning	32–39	.90
Supportive/protective/ corrective environment	40–49 (items 50 & 51 added after initial study)	.79
Human needs assistance	52–60	.89
Existential/phenomen- ological/spiritual forces	61–63	.66

Validity

Face and content validity were established by a panel of four content specialists familiar with Watson's conceptual model. The congruency of each behavior with its given subscale was rated by the panel and those items with interrater reliabilities of less than .75 were recategorized into more appropriate subscales.

Based on the results of the study described in the July/August, 1988 issue of *Heart and Lung*, two items were added to the Supportive/protective/ corrective environment subscale (Items 50 & 51). Reported alpha coefficients do not include these items.

7

Caring Behaviors of Nurses Scale

(Hinds, 1988)

The Caring Behaviors of Nurses Scale (CBNS) was developed by Hinds (1988) as a 22-item Visual Analogue Scale (VAS). The conceptual framework was derived from existential theory of nursing (humanistic nursing) (Paterson & Zderad, 1976). Such a perspective involves an intersubjective, nurse-patient relationship used to nurture the well-being and personal growth of patients (Hinds, 1988). While the theory guiding the tool was existential, the conceptual basis of caring behaviors on the CHNS was designed to detect nursing caring actions, as "the composite of purposeful nursing acts and attitudes which seek to 1) alleviate undue discomforts and meet anticipated needs of patients, 2) convey concern for the well-being of patients, and 3) communicate professional competence to patients" (Hinds, 1988; Beck, 1999).

The tool was developed to explore and describe the relationship of nurses' caring behaviors with hopefulness and health care outcomes in a group of adolescents receiving inpatient treatment for substance abuse. One of the unique features of the development of the CBNS was the relationship Hinds made between the abstract existential theory of humanistic (caring) relationship and the middle-range constructs derived from the theory. In her research with adolescents she made explicit the movement from abstract theory to middle-range constructs; she then theorized the relationships among study variables and anticipated findings. In developing and using the CBNS, the theory and middle-range constructs were translated into specific items. These items ultimately resulted in empirical measurements, based upon how closely each one indicated that "your thoughts about the actions of the nurse compare with those on the questionnaire," for example: "Nurses try to help me with worries"; "Nurses believe I can succeed"; "Nurses give me support when things go bad." Each item has a possible response range of 0–100 points. The higher the score, the higher the patients' perception of being cared for by the nurse. Hinds indicated that the CBNS had face and content validity, form equivalence, and internal consistency, based upon her earlier dissertation research (Hinds, 1985).

Hind's actual study testing the tool was a longitudinal, descriptive-correlational design, using both quantitative and qualitative methods to "systematically study the relationships specified in the conceptual framework, and to elicit information about change in each concept" (Hinds, 1988). The study design had three data collection points with 25 adolescents hospitalized in an inpatient substance abuse treatment unit in the Southwest. The first data collection: 24–28 hours after admission; Time 2: 96–120 hours before discharge; Time 3: 4–5 weeks after discharge from the unit. A Cronbach's alpha of 0.86 was reported for the CBNS for both Time 1 and Time 2. In addition to completing the visual analogue instruments, they also responded to a set of open-ended questions indexing the study concepts. The study using the CBNS provided "support for the theorized link between nurse-patient relationships and positive patient change" (Hinds, 1988). The instrument is copyrighted and the author requests that anyone wishing to use it, contact her. The matrix in Table 7.1 below includes the most salient features of the Caring Behaviors of Nurses Scale (CBNS).

TABLE 7.1 Matrix of Caring Behavior of Nurses Scale (Hinds, 1988)

Instrument & Year Developed	Author Contact Address	Year Published Source Citation	Developed to Measure	Instrument Description	Participants	Reported Reliability/Validity	Conceptual-Theoretical Basis of Measurement	Latest Citations in Nursing Literature
Caring Behaviors of Nurses Scale (CBNS) Hinds 1985, 1988	Pamela S. Hinds, RN, PhD, CS Director of Nursing Research, St. Jude Children's Research Hospital, 332 North Lauderdale, Memphis, TN 38105 Pam.Hinds@stjude.org	Hinds, P. S. (1988). The relationship of nurses' caring behaviors with hopefulness and health care outcomes in adolescents. *Archives of Psychiatric Nursing,* 2(1), 21–29.	Caring behaviors of nurses within intersubjective human relationship	Inductively based 22-item visual analogue scale, with possible range of 0 to 100 points; highest score, indicating perception of being more cared for by nurse	n = 25 Adolescent inpatients on substance abuse treatment unit in SW	Reported to have face and content validity, form equivalence, and internal consistency (Hinds, 1985); with adolescent study (1988) Cronbach's alpha of 0.86 for two data collection points; pragmatic content analysis and semantic content analysis achieved pre-established criterion levels of .8 or higher across the data collection points inter-coder reliability, stability	Existential-Humanistic Nursing (Paterson & Zderad) intersubjective relationship of caring	Hinds, 1988

CARING BEHAVIOR OF NURSES SCALE*

This questionnaire contains statements made by adolescents who are describing their thoughts about the actions or behaviors of the nurses who gave care to them. Please use this questionnaire to indicate how closely your thoughts about the actions of your nurses compare with those on this questionnaire. Because your answers are describing your honest opinions, there are no right or wrong answers. It is very important that you answer each statement according to your real opinion at this time.

Directions:

Beneath each statement is a line. On each end of the line is a phrase indicating how often the statement might be true for you. You may place an 'X' anywhere on the line between the two phrases to indicate how often your thoughts are like the thought expressed in the statement. Where you place your 'X' on the line does have meaning. The further to the left the 'X' is placed on the line, the less similar the statement is to your thoughts. The further to the right the 'X' is placed on the line, the more similar the statement is to your thoughts about nurses who gave care to you.

Here is an example:

A.   Nurses don't have patience with me.

NEVER TRUE FOR ME	X	X	X	ALWAYS TRUE FOR ME
	↑	↑	↑	
	If it is almost never true that your nurses don't have patience with you, your 'X' would be on the left part of the line.	If your nurses don't have patience with you about half the time, your 'X' would be about in the middle of the line.	If your nurses almost have no patience with you, your 'X' would be on the right side of the line.	

---

*©Pamela S. Hinds, RN, PhD, CS. Reprinted with permission of author.

THE CARING BEHAVIOR OF NURSES (FORM A)

1. Nurses try to help me with worries.
   NEVER TRUE   ALWAYS TRUE
   FOR ME   FOR ME

2. Nurses believe I can succeed.
   NEVER TRUE   ALWAYS TRUE
   FOR ME   FOR ME

3. Nurses point out positive things about me.
   NEVER TRUE   ALWAYS TRUE
   FOR ME   FOR ME

4. Nurses say I won't have a good future.
   NEVER TRUE   ALWAYS TRUE
   FOR ME   FOR ME

5. Nurses give me their suggestions.
   NEVER TRUE   ALWAYS TRUE
   FOR ME   FOR ME

6. Nurses are not interested in what I think.
   NEVER TRUE   ALWAYS TRUE
   FOR ME   FOR ME

7. Nurses tell me there is a chance if I try.
   NEVER TRUE   ALWAYS TRUE
   FOR ME   FOR ME

8. Nurses point out what things could happen to me in the future.
   NEVER TRUE   ALWAYS TRUE
   FOR ME   FOR ME

9. Nurses don't try to understand me.
   NEVER TRUE   ALWAYS TRUE
   FOR ME   FOR ME

10. When I am upset, nurses help me get my mind off bad things.
    NEVER TRUE   ALWAYS TRUE
    FOR ME   FOR ME

11. Nurses do not trust me.
    NEVER TRUE   ALWAYS TRUE
    FOR ME   FOR ME

12. Nurses talk to me about things I don't understand.
    NEVER TRUE   ALWAYS TRUE
    FOR ME   FOR ME

13. Nurses tell me I can pull myself out of it.
NEVER TRUE   ALWAYS TRUE
FOR ME   FOR ME

14. Nurses don't point out my progress.
NEVER TRUE   ALWAYS TRUE
FOR ME   FOR ME

15. Because of the nurses, I know I'm not alone.
NEVER TRUE   ALWAYS TRUE
FOR ME   FOR ME

16. Nurses don't support my efforts to get better.
NEVER TRUE   ALWAYS TRUE
FOR ME   FOR ME

17. Nurses are honest with me.
NEVER TRUE   ALWAYS TRUE
FOR ME   FOR ME

18. Nurses refuse to help me with my problems.
NEVER TRUE   ALWAYS TRUE
FOR ME   FOR ME

19. If nurses see what I don't see, they point it out to me.
NEVER TRUE   ALWAYS TRUE
FOR ME   FOR ME

20. Nurses tell me if I work at it, things will get better.
NEVER TRUE   ALWAYS TRUE
FOR ME   FOR ME

21. Nurses don't seem to care about my getting well.
NEVER TRUE   ALWAYS TRUE
FOR ME   FOR ME

22. Nurses believe I can change.
NEVER TRUE   ALWAYS TRUE
FOR ME   FOR ME

Thank you very much for participating!

THE CARING BEHAVIOR OF NURSES (FORM B)

1. Nurses talk with me about my problems.
NEVER TRUE   ALWAYS TRUE
FOR ME   FOR ME

2. The nurses believe in me.
    NEVER TRUE   ALWAYS TRUE
    FOR ME   FOR ME

3. Nurses point out good things about me.
    NEVER TRUE   ALWAYS TRUE
    FOR ME   FOR ME

4. Nurses tell me my future won't be good.
    NEVER TRUE   ALWAYS TRUE
    FOR ME   FOR ME

5. Nurses give me advice.
    NEVER TRUE   ALWAYS TRUE
    FOR ME   FOR ME

6. Nurses are not willIng to listen to me.
    NEVER TRUE   ALWAYS TRUE
    FOR ME   FOR ME

7. Nurses tell me life is worth it if I try.
    NEVER TRUE   ALWAYS TRUE
    FOR ME   FOR ME

8. Nurses point out what my future could be like.
    NEVER TRUE   ALWAYS TRUE
    FOR ME   FOR ME

9. Nurses don't show any interest in helping me.
    NEVER TRUE   ALWAYS TRUE
    FOR ME   FOR ME

10. Nurses give me support when things go bad.
    NEVER TRUE   ALWAYS TRUE
    FOR ME   FOR ME

11. Nurses don't let me make my own decisions.
    NEVER TRUE   ALWAYS TRUE
    FOR ME   FOR ME

12. Nurses explain things when I don't see why something happened.
    NEVER TRUE   ALWAYS TRUE
    FOR ME   FOR ME

13. Nurses tell me it's not useless.
    NEVER TRUE   ALWAYS TRUE
    FOR ME   FOR ME

14. Nurses don't point out positive change in me.
NEVER TRUE   ALWAYS TRUE
FOR ME   FOR ME

15. Nurses help by just being around.
NEVER TRUE   ALWAYS TRUE
FOR ME   FOR ME

16. I don't get help from the nurses.
NEVER TRUE   ALWAYS TRUE
FOR ME   FOR ME

17. I can believe what the nurses say to me.
NEVER TRUE   ALWAYS TRUE
FOR ME   FOR ME

18. Nurses won't listen to my problems.
NEVER TRUE   ALWAYS TRUE
FOR ME   FOR ME

19. Nurses point out things I hadn't thought of.
NEVER TRUE   ALWAYS TRUE
FOR ME   FOR ME

20. Nurses tell me something good will happen if I try to make things better.
NEVER TRUE   ALWAYS TRUE
FOR ME   FOR ME

21. Nurses don't seem hopeful for me to do well.
NEVER TRUE   ALWAYS TRUE
FOR ME   FOR ME

22. Nurses think there is hope for me.
NEVER TRUE   ALWAYS TRUE
FOR ME   FOR ME

Thank you very much for participating!

8

Professional Caring Behaviors

(Horner, 1989, 1991)

The Professional Caring Behaviors (PCB) would be considered a first generation measurement instrument. It was developed by Sharon Horner in 1989 and 1991 and was further refined by Harrison (1995). It was developed by having 356 patients respond to four open-ended questions about nurse caring behaviors. The process generated 28 items in two different forms (A & B). The total number of statements was 56, which included two positive statements, and two negative statements for each theme.

A 4-point Likert Scale was used, ranging from "strongly agree" to "strongly disagree." A panel of four nurse experts established content validity. Harrison used the instrument to compare perceptions of nurse caring behaviors of in-patient hospice nurses and the families of inpatient hospice clients. A convenience sample of 28 nurses and patient family members (14 each) on the inpatient hospice facility were used for establishing some of the psychometric characteristics of the instrument.

A test-retest reliability of .81 was reported (Harrison, 1995). Only one item, "The caring nurse respects the patient's spiritual beliefs," was significantly more important to the nurses than the family members, again highlighting a consistent finding across several studies and with use of different instruments (beginning with original work by Larson, 1984). A Cronbach's alpha of .92 for Form A and .94 for Form B was reported; Pearson's correlation between positive and negative statements was .00. Additional psychometric data can be obtained by communicating directly with Dr. Horner at the University of Texas at Austin.

The conceptual basis of the use of the instrument (Harrison, 1995) seemed to be guided by an interest in examining family perceptions of nurse caring, instead of usual patient or nurse perceptions. The conceptual-theoretical basis of the instrument is not made explicit, although general nursing theory and nursing literature and earlier research on caring is noted. The instrument is copyrighted and the author requests that she be contacted for its use. Table 8.1 below includes a matrix of the instrument: Professional Caring Behaviors (PCB).

TABLE 8.1 Matrix of Professional Caring Behaviors (Horner, 1991)

Instrument & Year Developed	Author Contact Address	Year Published Source Citation	Developed to Measure	Instrument Description	Participants	Reported Reliability/ Validity	Conceptual-Theoretical Basis of Measurement	Latest Citation of Instrument
Professional Caring Behaviors Horner, 1989, 1991	Sharon D. Horner, PhD, RN, University of Texas at Austin, 1700 Red River, Austin, TX 78701-1499 s.horner@ mail.utexas. edu	Personal communication only (Harrison, 1995 publication, see below)	Perceptions of nurse caring behaviors	4 open-ended questions Two Forms (A & B), 28 items each	Patients n = 356	Test-retest .81 Cronbach's alpha .92 & .94 Pearson r .001	None stated, but refers to general caring theory literature	Harrison, E. (1995) Nurse caring: The new health care paradigm. *Journal of Nursing Care Quality*, 9(4), 14–23.

TABLE 8.1 Matrix of Professional Caring Behaviors (Horner, 1991)

Instrument & Year Developed	Author Contact Address	Year Published Source Citation	Developed to Measure	Instrument Description	Participants	Reported Reliability/ Validity	Conceptual- Theoretical Basis of Measurement	Latest Citation of Instrument
Professional Caring Behaviors Horner, 1989, 1991	Sharon D. Horner, PhD, RN, University of Texas at Austin, 1700 Red River, Austin, TX 78701-1499 s.horner@ mail.utexas. edu	Personal communication only (Harrison, 1995 publication, see below)	Perceptions of nurse caring behaviors	4 open-ended questions Two Forms (A & B), 28 items each	Patients n = 356	Test-retest .81 Cronbach's alpha .92 & .94 Pearson r .001	None stated, but refers to general caring theory literature	Harrison, E. (1995) Nurse caring: The new health care paradigm. *Journal of Nursing Care Quality*, 9(4), 14–23.

PROFESSIONAL CARING BEHAVIORS*
FORM A

Completion of this tool implies consent has been given.

Age _____   Male _____   Female _____

Social Security Number: XXX-XX- __ __ __ __

Directions: Read each statement, then indicate the degree to which you agree or disagree that the statement indicates Professional Caring.

Strongly Disagree = SD   Disagree = D   Agree = A   Strongly Agree = SA

1. The caring nurse explains things in a way   SD   D   A   SA
    that is over the patient's head.
2. The caring nurse uses a gentle tone of voice   SD   D   A   SA
    during procedures.
3. The caring nurse takes a few minutes just to   SD   D   A   SA
    talk.
4. The caring nurse understands and shares in   SD   D   A   SA
    the patient's experiences.
5. The caring nurse is poorly organized when   SD   D   A   SA
    providing care.
6. The caring nurse touches patients roughly   SD   D   A   SA
    when they are hurting.
7. The caring nurse seems to be "going through   SD   D   A   SA
    the motions" without any real feeling.
8. The caring nurse straightens up patient   SD   D   A   SA
    rooms to look nicer.
9. The caring nurse enters rooms without   SD   D   A   SA
    knocking.
10. The caring nurse listens carefully to com-   SD   D   A   SA
    plaints.
11. The caring nurse learns of patient's special   SD   D   A   SA
    needs.
12. The caring nurse gives shots in a manner   SD   D   A   SA
    that causes patients less pain and stress.
13. The caring nurse speaks in a harsh manner.   SD   D   A   SA
14. The caring nurse expresses concern for pa-   SD   D   A   SA
    tients.

*©Copyright Horner, 1989. Reprinted with permission of author.

15.	The caring nurse does not show real interest in patient's problems.	SD D A SA
16.	The caring nurse takes time with patients' families.	SD D A SA
17.	The caring nurse does not attend to patients' spiritual beliefs.	SD D A SA
18.	The caring nurse remembers patients as real people.	SD D A SA
19.	The caring nurse is abrupt and hurried in completing work.	SD D A SA
20.	The caring nurses looks unfriendly at patients.	SD D A SA
21.	The caring nurse does not give information to patient's family.	SD D A SA
22.	The caring nurse is not concerned about patient problems.	SD D A SA
23.	The caring nurse leaves soiled linen and dressings in patient's rooms.	SD D A SA
24.	The caring nurse touches the patient appropriately.	SD D A SA
25.	The caring nurse gives carefully thought out answers.	SD D A SA
26.	The caring nurse respects patient's spiritual needs.	SD D A SA
27.	The caring nurse does not listen when patients talk about problems and concerns.	SD D A SA
28.	The caring nurse gives warm smiles.	SD D A SA

In the space below, describe other caring behaviors that come to mind.

PROFESSIONAL CARING BEHAVIORS
FORM B

Completion of this tool implies consent has been given.

Age _____   Male _____   Female _____

Social Security Number: XXX-XX- __ __ __ __

Directions: Read each statement, then indicate the degree to which you agree or disagree that the statement indicates Professional Caring.

Strongly Disagree = SD   Disagree = D   Agree = A   Strongly Agree = SA

1. The caring nurse does a procedure without SD D A SA
   an explanation.
2. The caring nurse leaves soiled equipment in SD D A SA
   the patient room.
3. The caring nurse's face reflects kindness and SD D A SA
   concern.
4. The caring nurse answers the call light in a SD D A SA
   short period of time.
5. The caring nurse is well organized. SD D A SA
6. The caring nurse treats patients like objects. SD D A SA
7. The caring nurse talks in a warm friendly SD D A SA
   manner.
8. The caring nurse gives support to patients' SD D A SA
   families.
9. The caring nurse gives opinions without re- SD D A SA
   gard for the patient's spiritual beliefs.
10. The caring nurse is concerned with patients' SD D A SA
    problems.
11. The caring nurse ignores patients when they SD D A SA
    are upset or crying.
12. The caring nurse shows interest when pa- SD D A SA
    tients describe problems.
13. The caring nurse answers before patients SD D A SA
    have finished talking.
14. The caring nurse takes a long time to bring SD D A SA
    pain medication.
15. The caring nurse finds some way to make SD D A SA
    the patients' room more pleasant.
16. The caring nurse moves patients roughly. SD D A SA
17. The caring nurse seldom smiles. SD D A SA
18. The caring nurse stays with patients who are SD D A SA
    experiencing discomfort.
19. The caring nurse does not look at patients SD D A SA
    while doing routine procedures.
20. The caring nurse listens to patients problems SD D A SA
    when they need to talk.
21. The caring nurse gives clear explanations SD D A SA
    about procedures, tests, and medicines.
22. The caring nurse ignores the patient's fam- SD D A SA
    ily.
23. The caring nurse touches patients in a sup- SD D A SA
    portive manner.

24. The caring nurse respects patient's spiritual   SD   D   A   SA
    beliefs.
25. The caring nurse speaks in a loud sharp   SD   D   A   SA
    voice.
26. The caring nurse has trouble managing   SD   D   A   SA
    equipment.
27. The caring nurse calls patients by their   SD   D   A   SA
    proper name.
28. The caring nurse does not appear concerned   SD   D   A   SA
    by patients' complaints.

In the space below, please describe the caring behaviors you remember
the most.

9

Nyberg Caring Assessment (Attributes) Scale

(Nyberg, 1990)

Nyberg's Caring Assessment (also referred to as Caring Attributes) Scale (CAS) was based upon caring attributes reported in the literature. She reports basing scale development on Watson and "theoretically related caring theorists," including Mayeroff and Noddings (Nyberg, 1990). Nyberg was interested in the relation between effects of caring and economics on nursing practice. It is interesting that her instrument is not focused on behavior, rather attributes, whereby she is attempting to philosophically and operationally capture the subjective aspect of caring. The caring attributes are such dimensions as deep respect for the needs of others, a belief that others have potential, and commitment to relationship. She focused on the human care element of nursing as part of the development. For example, items from the carative factors (Watson, 1979) are: helping/trusting relationship, understanding spiritual aspects, solving problems creatively, and being sensitive to self and others/sustaining hope.

The original instrument was formulated during her doctoral studies at the University of Colorado. The original questions for the instrument were derived directly from the literature [the first 7 items from the carative factors of Watson (1979, 1985); the others from Gaut (1983); Noddings (1984); and Mayeroff (1971)]. Three hundred and fifty questionnaires were sent to a random sample of nurses and 135 were returned. The overall population from which this random sample was drawn included 22,793 nurses from 7 hospitals.

The original developmental work resulted in a Cronbach's alpha of .80–.90. The actual study with the 135 returned questionnaires had an alpha of .85–.97. There is very little information available on construct validity. This instrument has potential for further use and refinement, but to date the use of the CAS has not been reported in additional research studies. The instrument is copyrighted and the author requests that she be contacted for permission and advice regarding its use. Table 9.1 below provides a matrix for Nyberg's caring attributes scale.

TABLE 9.1 Matrix for Nyberg Caring Attributes Scale (Nyberg, 1990)

Instrument & Year Developed	Author Contact Address	Year Published and Source Citation	Developed to Measure	Instrument Description	Participants	Reported Reliability/ Validity	Conceptual-Theoretical Basis of Measurement	Latest Citation in Nursing Literature
Nyberg Caring Attributes Scale (CAS) 1989, 1990	Jan Nyberg, RN, PhD, 13502 W. 63rd Place, Arvada, Colorado 80004 303-425-1219 jannyberg7 @aol.com	Nyberg, J. (1990). The effects of care and economics on nursing practice. *Journal of Nursing Administration,* 20(5), 13–18.	Caring attributes of nurses—more subjective human element, than behaviors	20 items, on five-point Likert scale; 4 separate rating scales on items	n = 135 nurses from random sample mailing of questionnaire	Cronbach's alpha reported at: .87–.98. No discussion of construct or content validity—except use of theory factors, previously tested (Cronin & Harrison, 1988)	Draws directly from caring theory literature, specific items from Watson's caring factors; others from Noddings, Gaut, Mayeroff	Nyberg, J. (1990). The effects of care and economics on nursing practice. *Journal of Nursing Administration,* 20(5), 13–18.

NYBERG CARING ASSESSMENT SCALE*

Are these caring attributes things you actually use in your day-to-day practice?

Always use in practice   5
Often use in practice   4
Sometimes use in practice   3
Occasionally use in practice   2
Cannot use in practice   1

Do you:

1. Have deep respect for the needs of others.
2. Not give up hope for others.
3. Remain sensitive to the needs of others.
4. Communicate a helping, trusting attitude toward others.
5. Express positive and negative feelings.
6. Solve problems creatively.
7. Understand that spiritual forces contribute to human care.
8. Consider relationships before rules.
9. Base decisions on what is best for the people involved.
10. Understand thoroughly what situations mean to people.
11. Go beyond the superficial to know people well.
12. Implement skills and techniques well.
13. Choose tactics that will accomplish goals.
14. Give full consideration to situational factors.
15. Focus on helping others to grow.
16. Take time for personal needs and growth.
17. Allow time for caring opportunities.
18. Remain committed to a continuing relationship.
19. Listen carefully and be open to feedback.
20. Believe that others have a potential that can be achieved.

*Reprinted with permission of author.
*©Copyright Nyberg.

10

Caring Ability Inventory

(Nkongho, 1990)

The Caring Ability Inventory (CAI) was developed by Nkongho (1990) to measure one's ability to care when involved in a relationship with others. The conceptual basis for the instrument was derived from caring literature and the author's identification of four theoretical assumptions: 1) caring is multidimensional (with attitudinal and cognitive components); 2) the potential to care is present in all individuals; 3) caring can be learned; and 4) caring is quantifiable. Other aspects of caring are drawn upon as background for the instrument, but the more direct conceptual influence was Mayeroff's (1971) view of caring: "helping another to grow and actualize himself (sic) . . . and process, a way of relating to someone that involves development." Other indicators of caring, from Mayeroff, which informed the developments of the instrument are knowing, alternating rhythm, patience, honesty, trust, humility, hope, and courage (Nkongho, 1990).

During the early developmental stages of CAI, Mayeroff's framework was used to formulate the original items. They then were derived in two ways: review of caring literature, yielding 61 items from literature; and by developing 10 open-ended questions, that were asked of 15 consenting adults. From these 15 adult interviews, 19 additional items were derived and a total of 80 items were constructed for the first version: 34 positive statements and 46 negative statements. The 80 items were placed on a 7-point Likert scale.

The 80-item version was subjected to additional testing with the use of 543 participants and factor analysis of the items. From this process, subscales emerged that capture aspects such as knowing, courage, and patience, which are congruent with Mayeroff's theory. Each of the subscales has a number of items: Knowing = 14 items; Courage = 13 items; Patience = 10 items. The final version of the CAI consists of 37 items representing three of Mayeroff's theoretical elements of caring. Item responses are summed for each subscale, yielding a total score for each subscale. The higher scores indicate greater degree of caring if the item is positively phrased; scoring is reversed if the item is negatively worded.

Additional reliability and validity was assessed through Cronbach's alphas and test-retest administration (after a two-week period). The alpha coefficient for each of the subscales ranged from .71–.84 (n = 537); the test-retest r ranged from .64–.80 (n = 38).

Content validity was established through use of two experts in content area. Revisions were made and resubmitted to content reviewers, resulting in a content validity index (CVI), using the method outlined by Waltz & Strickland and Lenz (1984). The CVI was reported as .80. Construct validity was established by correlation with the Tennessee Self-Concept Scale as well as discrimination between groups (practicing nurses and college students; and female and male participants). The *t*-test on mean scores of groups were both statistically significant.

The various reliability and validity tests indicate the CAI is both reliable and valid for measuring caring elements of knowing, courage, and patience. As a self-report measure, the CAI is easy to administer and may be used for different professional groups (e.g., engineers, social workers, physicians, and nurses). Identifying individuals on the high or low dimensions of caring serves as a guide for counseling, guidance, and self-growth. The CAI has the potential for use in both academic and clinical settings.

The CAI has sophisticated psychometric properties that support its use and that help to assure its measurement confidence. The latest citation of the CAI noted in the health professional literature was a research study by Simmons and Cavanaugh (2000). They used the CAI in a study that examined the relationships among students and graduate's caring ability and school climate.

The CAI is copyrighted by Springer Publishing Company, 536 Broadway, New York, NY 10012-3955, telephone (212) 432-4370. Dr. Nkongho requests that anyone using the instrument contact her so that she can be informed as to its use, and be assisted in further refining the tool. Table 10.1 provides a matrix of contact information, properties of the CAI, and background data regarding its development.

TABLE 10.1 Matrix of Caring Ability Inventory (Nyongho, 1990)

Instrument & Year Developed	Author & Contact Address	Publication Source Citation	Developed to Measure	Instrument Description	Participants	Reported Reliability/Validity	Conceptual-Theoretical Basis of Measurement	Latest Citation in Nursing Literature
Caring Ability Inventory (CAI)	Ngozi O. Nkongho, RN, PhD Assistant Professor, Lehman College, Department of Nursing, The City University of New York, New York, NY Ph: 718.960.8794 *ngozi@alpha.lehman.cuny.edu*	Nkongho, N. (1990). The Caring Ability Inventory. In *Measurement of Nursing Outcomes. Vol. 4*, O. L. Strickland & C. R. Waltz (Eds.). New York: Springer. 3–13; 14–16.	Ones' ability to care (when involved in relationship)	Self-administered 7-point Likert; 47 items; 3 major factors: knowing, courage, patience; measured with subscales	n = 462 college students, varied majors; n = 75 nurses (attending professional conference)	Cronbach's alpha for each factor (.71–.84 range) Factor Analysis for collapsing items Test-Retest r = .64–.80 range content validity with experts; construct validity between group discrimination and correlation with Tennessee Self-Concept Scale	General review of caring theory literature; specific development informed by Mayeroff's eight critical elements of caring	Nkongho, N. (1990). The Caring Ability Inventory. In *Measurement of Nursing Outcomes. Vol. 4.* O. L. Strickland & C. R. Waltz (Eds.) New York: Springer. 3–13; 14–16. Cavanaugh, S., & Simmons, P. (1997). Evaluation of a school climate for assessing af-

TABLE 10.1 *(continued)*

Instrument & Year Developed	Author & Contact Address	Publication Source Citation	Developed to Measure	Instrument Description	Participants	Reported Reliability/Validity	Conceptual-Theoretical Basis of Measurement	Latest Citation in Nursing Literature
								fective objectives in health professional education. *Evaluation and the Health Professions, 20*(4), 455–478. Simmons, P. R., & Cavanaugh, S. H. (2000). Relationships among student and graduate caring ability and professional school climate. *Journal of Professional Nursing, 16*(2), 76–83.

CARING ABILITY INVENTORY*

Please read each of the following statements and decide how well it reflects your thoughts and feelings about other people in general. There is no right or wrong answer. Using the response scale, from 1 to 7, circle the degree to which you agree or disagree with each statement directly on the booklet. Please answer all questions.

1   2   3   4   5   6   7

strongly   strongly
disagree   agree

		Strongly Disagree					Strongly Agree	
		1	2	3	4	5	6	7
1.	I believe that learning takes time.	1	2	3	4	5	6	7
2.	Today is filled with opportunities.	1	2	3	4	5	6	7
3.	I usually say what I mean to others.	1	2	3	4	5	6	7
4.	There is very little I can do for a person who is helpless.	1	2	3	4	5	6	7
5.	I can see the need for change in myself.	1	2	3	4	5	6	7
6.	I am able to like people even if they don't like me.	1	2	3	4	5	6	7
7.	I understand people easily.	1	2	3	4	5	6	7
8.	I have seen enough in this world for what I need to know.	1	2	3	4	5	6	7
9.	I make the time to get to know other people.	1	2	3	4	5	6	7
10.	Sometimes I like to be involved and sometimes I do not like being involved.	1	2	3	4	5	6	7
11.	There is nothing I can do to make life better.	1	2	3	4	5	6	7
12.	I feel uneasy knowing that another person depends on me.	1	2	3	4	5	6	7
13.	I do not like to go out of my way to help other people.	1	2	3	4	5	6	7
14.	In dealing with people, it is difficult to let my feelings show.	1	2	3	4	5	6	7

*Reprinted with permission of Springer Publishing.

15.	It does not matter what I say, as long as I do the correct thing.	1	2	3	4	5	6	7
16.	I find it difficult to understand how the other person feels if I have not had similar experiences.	1	2	3	4	5	6	7
17.	I admire people who are calm, composed, and patient.	1	2	3	4	5	6	7
18.	I believe it is important to accept and respect the attitudes and feelings of others.	1	2	3	4	5	6	7
19.	People can count on me to do what I say I will.	1	2	3	4	5	6	7
20.	I believe that there is room for improvement.	1	2	3	4	5	6	7
21.	Good friends look after each other.	1	2	3	4	5	6	7
22.	I find meaning in every situation.	1	2	3	4	5	6	7
23.	I am afraid to "let go" of those I care for because I am afraid of what might happen to them.	1	2	3	4	5	6	7
24.	I like to offer encouragement to people.	1	2	3	4	5	6	7
25.	I do not like to make commitments beyond the present.	1	2	3	4	5	6	7
26.	I really like myself.	1	2	3	4	5	6	7
27.	I see strengths and weaknesses (limitations) in each individual.	1	2	3	4	5	6	7
28.	New experiences are usually frightening to me.	1	2	3	4	5	6	7
29.	I am afraid to be open and let others see who I am.	1	2	3	4	5	6	7
30.	I accept people just the way they are.	1	2	3	4	5	6	7
31.	When I care for someone else, I do not have to hide my feelings.	1	2	3	4	5	6	7
32.	I do not like to be asked for help.	1	2	3	4	5	6	7
33.	I can express my feelings to people in a warm and caring way.	1	2	3	4	5	6	7
34.	I like talking with people.	1	2	3	4	5	6	7
35.	I regard myself as sincere in my relationships with others.	1	2	3	4	5	6	7
36.	People need space (room, privacy) to think and feel.	1	2	3	4	5	6	7
37.	I can be approached by people at any time.	1	2	3	4	5	6	7

SCORING INFORMATION

Items to be summed for each subscale:

Knowing: 2, 3, 6, 7, 9, 19, 22, 26, 30, 31, 33, 34, 35, 36.
Courage: 4, 8, 11, 12, 13, 14, 15, 16, 23, 25, 28, 29, 32.
Patience: 1, 5, 10, 17, 18, 20, 21, 24, 27, 36.
Items to be reverse-scored: 4, 8, 11, 12, 13, 14, 15, 16, 23, 25, 28, 29, 32.

The nurse group comprised 75 practicing nurses attending a national conference. Participants came from all areas of the country. To determine ranges for low, medium, and high norm scores, .5 standard deviation on either side of the mean was considered to be in the middle range of scores. Scores above this were considered high, and scores below this were considered low. See Table 1.8 for low, medium, and high norms for the nurse group.

The college students group consisted of 424 females and 103 males attending a large university in metropolitan New York. The students represented a wide variety of ability, ethnic, and socioeconomic groups. Low, medium, and high groups were determined in the same way as above. See Table 1.9 for low, medium, and high norms for female and male college students.

Low, Medium, High Norms for CAI and Its Subscales for Nurses

Subscale	Low	Medium	High
Knowing	Below 76.4	76.4–84.0	Above 84.0
Courage	Below 62.5	62.5–74.0	Above 74.0
Patience	Below 61.0	61.0–65.2	Above 65.2
Total CAI	Below 203.1	203.1–220.3	Above 220.3

Low, Medium, High Norms for CAI and Its Subscales for Female and Male College Students

Subscale	Females ($n = 424$)			Males ($n = 103$)		
	Low	Medium	High	Low	Medium	High
Knowing	< 68.8	68.8–79.5	> 79.5	< 64.6	64.6–75.1	> 75.11
Courage	< 62.14	62.14–73.06	> 73.06	< 54.41	54.41–66.56	> 66.56
Patience	< 58.05	58.05–64.35	> 64.35	< 53.4	53.4–62.4	> 62.4
Total CAI	< 190.29	190.29–211.12	> 211.12	< 178.00	178.00–199.36	> 199.36

11

Caring Behavior Checklist and Client Perception of Caring

(McDaniel, 1990)

These two measures, the Caring Behavior Checklist (CBC) and the Client Perception of Caring (CPC) were developed by McDaniel to measure caring behaviors of nurses as they care for clients. As part of the conceptual background for the instrument's development, McDaniel (1990) distinguished between the notions of *caring for* and *caring about*. The process of caring (which involves *caring about*) was conceptualized at four levels:

- Acknowledgement of need for care (involves existential I-Thou relationship)
- Decision to care (involves commitment on behalf of well-being of other)
- Actions (acts and behaviors intended to promote welfare of other—external manifestations of internal processes)
- Actualization (ultimate result of caring process and perception of other as being cared for and about—satisfaction in both nurse and other).

In developing the instruments, caring behaviors were defined as those verbal and nonverbal actions denoting care performed by the nurse—this was operational based upon the subjective and affective responses of clients to nurses' caring behaviors. The Caring Behavior Checklist was designed to measure the presence or absence of specific actions denoting care, not to quantify the degree or amount of care (McDaniel, 1990). The Client Perception of Caring is a questionnaire designed to measure the client's response to the caring behaviors of the nurse. The items for the second instrument were developed from studies which described reactions of clients to nurse-client interactions, in order to get at the more essential structure of the caring interaction as experienced by the client.

The two instruments are designed to be used together to capture the caring process. They are both intended for hospital setting use and administration. The CBC consists of 12 items that represent caring behaviors; its use requires a trained observer to score a nurse-client interaction for a period of 30 minutes and each behavior is dichotomously scored as either present or absent. The range of scores is from 0 to 12; high scores indicate high numbers of behaviors were reportedly observed; low scores indicate few.

The Client Perception of Caring (CPC) is administered to the client after the observation period. This tool has 10 items on a 6-point rating scale; each item is summed to obtain the score. The potential range of scores is from 10 to 60, with high indicating a high degree of caring as perceived by client, and low, indicating low caring behavior perceived by client.

Both reliability and validity were established for both instruments. Content validity was calculated for the Caring Behaviors Checklist as .80, using the content validity index (CVI) described by Waltz, Strickland, and Lenz (1984). Reliability of the Client Perception of Caring was established with internal consistency, with standardized item alpha calculated at .81. Item to total correlation averaged .41. Reliability for the CBC was through interrater agreements. Two trained raters scored the items independently and simultaneously on each of the 21 interactions. Agreements of each of the 12 items ranged from .76 to 1.00, with 8 of the 12 items having .90 or above rating scores. Efforts to estimate construct validity by correlating COC against the Empathy Scale (La Monica, 1981) was not conclusive, possibly due to the low number of subjects. The two instruments used together have promise in capturing both external behaviors as well as client perceptions around a shared caring occasion. Additional research is recommended with instrument refinement increasing potential for item variability on CBC. The instruments are copyrighted by Springer Publishing Company, 536 Broadway, New York, NY 10012-3955, Telephone (212) 431-4370. Table 11.1 outlines in matrix format the key properties of both instruments.

TABLE 11.1 Matrix of Caring Behaviors Checklist and Client Perception of Caring (McDaniel, 1990)

Instrument and Year Developed	Author & Contact Address	Publication Source Citation	Developed to Measure	Instrument Description	Participants	Reported Reliability/ Validity	Conceptual- Theoretical Basis of Measurement	Latest Citation in Nursing Literature
Caring Behaviors Checklist (CBC)	Anna McDaniel, RN, CS, MA. Last Contact Address: Assistant Professor of Nursing Education, Division of Nursing, Indiana Wesleyan University, Marion, Indiana **(unable to obtain current contact address)**	McDaniel, A. M. (1990). The caring process in nursing: Two instruments for measuring caring behaviors. In *Measurement of Nursing Outcomes.* Strickland, O., & Waltz, C. (Eds.). New York: Springer: 17–27.	Caring process (external observable)	12 items of observable caring behaviors; dichotomous scoring of each item by trained observer(s)	Junior Nursing Student—patient interactions n = not given	Interrater reliability, 92 overall on 12 items; Content Validity Index (CVI) .80	Informed by philosophical views in general caring literature; interest in *caring about* as well as *caring for,* guided instrument development	McDaniel, A. M. (1990). The caring process in nursing: Two instruments for measuring caring behaviors. In *Measurement of Nursing Outcomes.* Strickland, O., & Waltz, C. (Eds.). New York: Springer.

(continued)

TABLE 11.1 *(continued)*

Instrument and Year Developed	Author & Contact Address	Publication Source Citation	Developed to Measure	Instrument Description	Participants	Reported Reliability/ Validity	Conceptual-Theoretical Basis of Measurement	Latest Citation in Nursing Literature
Client Perception of Caring Scale (CPC)	McDaniel, A. M. (see above)	Citation above	Clients' perception of nurse caring (detect both caring and non-caring behaviors as perceived by clients)	Designed to be used with CBC in hospital setting 10 items rated on 6-point scale; Scores range from 10–60	Number of participants not given; junior-level nursing students in BS nursing program	Content Validity 1.00 using CVI Alpha .81 reliability; item to total correlation .41 Construct validity not significant after correction with Empathy scale	General caring theory literature; Conceptual model of caring process developed to guide instrument	McDaniel, A. M. (1990). The caring process in nursing: Two instruments for measuring caring behaviors. In *Measurement of Nursing Outcomes*. Strickland, O., & Waltz, C. (Eds.) New York: Springer.

CARING BEHAVIOR CHECKLIST AND CLIENT PERCEPTION OF CARING SCALE*

CARING BEHAVIOR CHECKLIST

Absent = 0
Present = 1

Verbal Caring Behaviors

Verbally responds to an expressed concern.
Explains procedure prior to initiation.
Verbally validates patient's physical status.
Verbally validates patient's emotional status.
Shares personal observations or feelings (self-disclosing)
    in response to patient's expression of concern.
Verbally reassures patient during care.
Discusses topics of patients concern other than current
    health problems.

Nonverbal Caring Behaviors

Sits down at bedside.
Touches patient exclusive of procedure.
Sustains eye contact during patient interaction.
Enters patient room without solicitation.
Provides physical comfort measures.

CLIENT PERCEPTION OF CARING SCALE

1. I felt that this nurse really listened to what I was saying.

/____1____/____2____/____3____/____4____/____5____/____6____/
Not at all   Very Much

2. I felt reassured when this nurse cared for me.

/____1____/____2____/____3____/____4____/____5____/____6____/
Not at all   Very Much

3. I felt that this nurse really valued me as an individual.

/____1____/____2____/____3____/____4____/____5____/____6____/
Not at all   Very Much

4. I felt free to talk to this nurse about what concerned me.

/____1____/____2____/____3____/____4____/____5____/____6____/
Not at all   Very Much

5. I felt the nurse was more interested in her "job" than my needs.

/____1____/____2____/____3____/____4____/____5____/____6____/
Not at all   Very Much

6. I felt that this nurse could tell when something was bothering me.

/____1____/____2____/____3____/____4____/____5____/____6____/
Not at all   Very Much

7. I felt secure with this nurse taking care of me.

/____1____/____2____/____3____/____4____/____5____/____6____/
Not at all   Very Much

8. I felt frustrated by this nurse's attitude.

/____1____/____2____/____3____/____4____/____5____/____6____/
Not at all   Very Much

9. I could tell this nurse really cared about me.

/____1____/____2____/____3____/____4____/____5____/____6____/
Not at all   Very Much

10. I could tell that this nurse wanted to make me feel comfortable.

/____1____/____2____/____3____/____4____/____5____/____6____/
Not at all   Very Much

12

Caring Assessment Tools

(Duffy, 1992, 2001)

Duffy developed the Caring Assessment Tool (CAT) for purposes of measuring nurse caring activities, as perceived by patients. It was constructed during the author's doctoral study (Duffy, 1990), and was designed to be used in a descriptive, correlational research design. Additional motivation for the tool's development was to establish a theoretically based and reliable instrument for use in a diverse patient population. The conceptual-theoretical basis for the instrument is derived from Watson's Caring Theory and attempts to measure the 10 carative factors that are embedded in the theory (Watson, 1979, 1985). It is suggested that the CAT is appropriate for formally researching nurse caring behaviors and outcomes of nursing care, via empirical measurements of the carative factors per se, as a test of the theory and as a validation of outcomes.

The instrument consists of 100 items on the Likert Scale ranging from 1 (low caring) to 5 (high caring) with a possible score range of 100–500. It is designed to be used with adult patients. The original development of the instrument used a sample of 86 patients with a medical-surgical diagnosis (Duffy, 1992). Psychometric properties of the CAT were not included in the published citation of the study, but noted that the information is available in the original dissertation, and/or by contacting the author of the tool directly.

Since the original CAT was developed, a 1993 CAT-admin version has evolved. The CAT-admin was designed to reflect staff nurses' perceptions of their managers for administrative nursing research. A qualitative question was added to the original tool to expand and enrich data collection. Like the original tool, Watson's carative factors were the theoretical basis for item development on the CAT-admin. A sample of 56 full- and part-time nurses were used in the tool revision. A Cronbach's alpha of .98 was reported for internal consistency. The author indicates the instruments are valid and reliable. Stepwise multiple regression was used to clarify the interrelationships between such variable as unit type, number of employees, and nursing turnover. In both Duffy's 1992 and 1993 citation of the tools' use, study results have reported a correlation between caring and patient satisfaction (CAT), and a correlation between nurse manager caring and staff nurse satisfaction (CAT-admin).

Duffy has recently developed a third version of the CAT, designed for nursing educational use, called the CAT-edu. It has not been published at this point, and is undergoing further refinement. This educational version of the caring instrument was tested on a convenience sample of 71 baccalaureate and master's nursing students. Internal consistency reliability data resulted in a Cronbach's alpha of .98 (Duffy, 2001, personal communication). The CAT-edu consists of a 5-point Likert-type scale, similar to the other versions, and has 95 items constructed for educational use. This instrument was adapted to measure students' perceptions of faculty caring behaviors. A copy of the CAT-edu instrument is included in the appendix.

These three versions of the Caring Assessment Tool (CAT, CAT-admin, and CAT-edu) are copyrighted by the author (Duffy, 1992, 1993, 2001). Anyone wishing to use these tools is encouraged to contact the developer directly for additional information and permission for use. Table 12.1 presents a matrix of key data related to the CAT, CAT-admin, and CAT-edu.

TABLE 12.1 Caring Assessment Tools, Caring Assessment Tool—Administrator Form, and Caring Assessment Tool—Educational Form (Duffy, 2000)

Instrument and Year Developed	Author & Contact Address	Year Publication Source Citation	Developed to Measure	Instrument Description	Participants	Reported Reliability/ Validity	Conceptual-Theoretical Basis of Measurement	Latest Citation in Nursing Literature
Caring Assessment Tool (CAT) ©Duffy 1990, 1992	Duffy, J. DNS Associate Professor of Nursing, Catholic University of America, Washington, DC 20064 202-319 6466 Duffy@cua.edu	Duffy, J. (1992). The impact of nurse caring on patient outcomes. In D. Gaut (Ed.), *The Presence of Caring in Nursing.* New York: NLN:113–136.	Patients' perception of nurse caring behaviors	100 items 5-point Likert	Medical-Surgical Patients n = 86	Internal consistency, test-retest reliability established; content validity reported in Duffy, 1990, dissertation work	Watson's theory of human caring; 10 carative factors	Duffy, J. (1993). Caring behaviors of nurse managers: Relationship to staff nurse satisfaction & retention. In Gaut, D., *A Global Agenda for Caring.* New York: NLN:365–378.

(continued)

127

TABLE 12.1 (*continued*)

Instrument and Year Developed	Author & Contact Address	Year Publication Source Citation	Developed to Measure	Instrument Description	Participants	Reported Reliability/Validity	Conceptual-Theoretical Basis of Measurement	Latest Citation in Nursing Literature
Caring Assessment Tool (Administrator Form) CAT-admin ©Duffy (1992, 1993)	See above	Duffy, J. (1993). Caring behaviors of nurse managers: Relationship to staff nurse satisfaction & retention. In Gaut, D., A Global Agenda for Caring. New York: NLN:365–378.	CAT-admin. Modified for nurses perception of nurse managers' caring behaviors; Relationship between staff nurse satisfaction & nurse managers' caring	94 items 5-point Likert	Nurses n = 56	See CAT, above & contact author	Watson's Theory and carative factors	See above
Caring Assessment Tool CAT-edu, Educational form of CAT ©Duffy, 2001	Duffy, 2001 See above	No publication source citation at this time	Educational version of CAT, focus on assessing students' perceptions of caring	5-point Likert scale; 95 items	n = 71 nursing students; baccalaureate and master's level	Earlier validity established; new Reliability on CAT-edu alpha = .9812	Original theory and conceptual basis: Watson Caring theory and Carative Factors	No publication to date on CAT-edu

CARING ASSESSMENT TOOL; CAT-ADMIN; CAT-EDU*

Code No. _____ (1–4)
Card No. _____ (5)

PATIENT SURVEY
CAT*

Directions: All of the statements in this survey refer to nursing activities that occur in a hospital. There are five possible responses to each item. They are:

1 = Never
2 = Rarely
3 = Occasionally
4 = Frequently
5 = Always

For each statement, please circle how often you think each activity is occurring during your hospitalization.

Since I have been a patient here, the nurses:

1. Listen to me. (6)
   1   2   3   4   5

2. Accept me as I am. (7)
   1   2   3   4   5

3. Treat me kindly. (8)
   1   2   3   4   5

4. Ignore me. (9)
   1   2   3   4   5

5. Answer my questions. (10)
   1   2   3   4   5

6. Include me in their discussions. (11)
   1   2   3   4   5

---

*©Jeanne R. Duffy. Reprinted by permission of author.
*©Joanne R. Duffy, R.N., D.N.Sc., (1990), Georgetown University School of Nursing, Washington, D.C.

Since I have been a patient here, the nurses:

7. Respect me.   (12)
   1   2   3   4   5

8. Are more interested in their own problems.   (13)
   1   2   3   4   5

9. Pay attention to me.   (14)
   1   2   3   4   5

10. Enjoy taking care of me.   (15)
    1   2   3   4   5

11. Use my name when they talk to me.   (16)
    1   2   3   4   5

12. Are available to me.   (17)
    1   2   3   4   5

13. Have no time for me.   (18)
    1   2   3   4   5

14. Seem interested in me.   (19)
    1   2   3   4   5

15. Support my sense of hope.   (20)
    1   2   3   4   5

16. Help me to believe in myself.   (21)
    1   2   3   4   5

17. Provide me with information.   (22)
    1   2   3   4   5

18. Fail to keep their promises to me.   (23)
    1   2   3   4   5

19. Encourage me to take care of myself.   (24)
    1   2   3   4   5

20. Support me with my beliefs.   (25)
    1   2   3   4   5

21. Encourage me to ask questions.   (26)
    1   2   3   4   5

22. Help me see some good aspects of my situation.   (27)
    1   2   3   4   5

Since I have been a patient here, the nurses:

23. Restrict my need for spiritual support. (28)
    1   2   3   4   5

24. Encourage my ability to go on with life. (29)
    1   2   3   4   5

25. Anticipate my needs. (30)
    1   2   3   4   5

26. Allow me to choose the best time to talk about my concerns. (31)
    1   2   3   4   5

27. Openly show concern for me. (32)
    1   2   3   4   5

28. Are concerned about my family's reaction to my illness. (33)
    1   2   3   4   5

29. Never show any emotion. (34)
    1   2   3   4   5

30. Ask me how I like things done. (35)
    1   2   3   4   5

31. Help me deal with my bad feelings. (36)
    1   2   3   4   5

32. When appropriate, share personal information with me. (37)
    1   2   3   4   5

33. Express human emotions when they are with me. (38)
    1   2   3   4   5

34. Respond honestly to my questions. (39)
    1   2   3   4   5

35. Initiate conversations with me. (40)
    1   2   3   4   5

36. Do not judge me. (41)
    1   2   3   4   5

37. Check on me frequently. (42)
    1   2   3   4   5

38. Look me in the eye when they talk to me. (43)
    1   2   3   4   5

39. Refuse to tell me aspects about my illness when I ask. (44)
    1   2   3   4   5

Since I have been a patient here, the nurses:

40. Pay attention to me when I am talking.   (45)
    1   2   3   4   5

41. Are responsive to my family.   (46)
    1   2   3   4   5

42. Act as if they disapprove of me.   (47)
    1   2   3   4   5

43. Talk openly to my family.   (48)
    1   2   3   4   5

44. Encourage me to talk about whatever is on my mind.   (49)
    1   2   3   4   5

45. Are patient with me even when I am difficult.   (50)
    1   2   3   4   5

46. Are interested in information I have to offer about my illness.   (51)
    1   2   3   4   5

47. Talk about me openly in front of other patients.   (52)
    1   2   3   4   5

48. Accept what I say, even if it is negative.   (53)
    1   2   3   4   5

49. Seem annoyed if I speak my true feelings.   (54)
    1   2   3   4   5

50. Are aware of my feelings.   (55)
    1   2   3   4   5

51. Do not want to talk to me.   (56)
    1   2   3   4   5

52. Allow me to talk about my true feelings without any risk to   (57)
    my care.
    1   2   3   4   5

53. Question me about my health history.   (58)
    1   2   3   4   5

54. Help me set health goals which I am able to do.   (59)
    1   2   3   4   5

55. Help me find solutions regarding my problems.   (60)
    1   2   3   4   5

Since I have been a patient here, the nurses:

56. Deal with my health problem in ways that are impractical for (61)
    me.
    1   2   3   4   5

57. Help me with all of my health problem/s, not just part of it. (62)
    1   2   3   4   5

58. Help me deal with difficult situations. (63)
    1   2   3   4   5

59. Help me understand how I am thinking about my illness. (64)
    1   2   3   4   5

60. Ask me how I think my hospitalization is going. (65)
    1   2   3   4   5

61. Help me explore alternative ways of dealing with my health (66)
    problem/s.
    1   2   3   4   5

62. Ask me what I know about my illness. (67)
    1   2   3   4   5

63. Provide me with literature about my illness. (68)
    1   2   3   4   5

64. Use medical terms that I don't understand. (69)
    1   2   3   4   5

65. Teach me how to care for myself. (70)
    1   2   3   4   5

66. Help me to figure out questions to ask my physician. (71)
    1   2   3   4   5

67. Discourage me from asking questions. (72)
    1   2   3   4   5

68. Check with me to make sure I understand what is happening (73)
    to me.
    1   2   3   4   5

69. Help me understand how my illness may affect my sexuality. (74)
    1   2   3   4   5

70. Make me feel as comfortable as possible. (75)
    1   2   3   4   5

Since I have been a patient here, the nurses:

71. Respect my need for privacy.   (76)
     1   2   3   4   5

72. Make sure the other nurses know how to take care of me.   (77)
     1   2   3   4   5

73. Know what to do in an emergency.   (78)
     1   2   3   4   5

74. Never ask what I need.   (79)
     1   2   3   4   5

75. Protect me from situations where I could get harmed.   (80)
     1   2   3   4   5

                                        Code No. _____ (1–4)
                                        Card No. _____ (5)

76. Encourage me to have personal items brought in from home.   (6)
     1   2   3   4   5

77. Know a lot about my health problem/s.   (7)
     1   2   3   4   5

78. Spend quiet time with me.   (8)
     1   2   3   4   5

79. Make me feel safe.   (9)
     1   2   3   4   5

80. Allow my family to visit often.   (10)
     1   2   3   4   5

81. Limit or interfere with my basic routine practices.   (11)
     1   2   3   4   5

82. Make sure I get the food I need.   (12)
     1   2   3   4   5

83. Give me good physical care.   (13)
     1   2   3   4   5

84. Monitor my activity level.   (14)
     1   2   3   4   5

85. Help me with my special routine needs for sleep.   (15)
     1   2   3   4   5

Since I have been a patient here, the nurses:

86. Make me wait a long time when I need help with bathroom (16)
   activities.
   1   2   3   4   5

87. Help me with my personal routines for bathing. (17)
   1   2   3   4   5

88. Help me feel less worried. (18)
   1   2   3   4   5

89. Allow me to be alone with my spouse and special family/ (19)
   friends.
   1   2   3   4   5

90. Discourage me from interacting with others. (20)
   1   2   3   4   5

91. Help me achieve my health goals. (21)
   1   2   3   4   5

92. Don't care how much I eat or drink. (22)
   1   2   3   4   5

93. Respect my need to sleep. (23)
   1   2   3   4   5

94. Understand my unique situation. (24)
   1   2   3   4   5

95. Have no idea how this illness is affecting my life. (25)
   1   2   3   4   5

96. Are concerned about how I view things. (26)
   1   2   3   4   5

97. Know what is important to me. (27)
   1   2   3   4   5

98. Acknowledge my inner feelings. (28)
   1   2   3   4   5

99. Help me cope with the stress of my illness. (29)
   1   2   3   4   5

Since I have been a patient here, the nurses:

100. Show respect for those things that have meaning to me.   (30)
         1   2   3   4   5

THIS IS THE END OF THE SURVEY. IF YOU WERE ASKED TO ADVISE
NURSES ON WHAT THEY NEED TO DO DIFFERENTLY, WHAT WOULD
YOU ADVISE? YOU MAY WRITE ON THE BACK OF THIS PAGE. THANK
YOU VERY MUCH FOR YOUR PARTICIPATION.

Code No. _____ (1–4)
Card No. _____ (5)

STAFF NURSE SURVEY
CAT-ADM*

Directions: All of the statements in this questionnaire refer to activities that occur among people on a nursing unit. There are five possible responses to each item. They are:

1 = Never
2 = Rarely
3 = Occasionally
4 = Frequently
5 = Always

For each statement, please circle how often you think each activity is occurring in your situation.

Since I have been a staff nurse here, my head nurse:

1. Listens to me. (6)
    1   2   3   4   5

2. Accepts me as I am. (7)
    1   2   3   4   5

3. Treats me kindly. (8)
    1   2   3   4   5

4. Ignores me. (9)
    1   2   3   4   5

5. Answers my questions. (10)
    1   2   3   4   5

6. Includes me in his/her discussions. (11)
    1   2   3   4   5

---

*©Joanne R. Duffy, D.N.Sc., R.N., CCRN, 1990, Georgetown University School of Nursing, Washington, D.C.
Reprinted with permission of author.

Since I have been a patient here, the nurses:

7. Respects me.   (12)
    1   2   3   4   5

8. Is more interested in his/her own problems.   (13)
    1   2   3   4   5

9. Pays attention to me.   (14)
    1   2   3   4   5

10. Enjoys working with me.   (15)
    1   2   3   4   5

11. Uses my name when talking to me.   (16)
    1   2   3   4   5

12. Is available to me.   (17)
    1   2   3   4   5

13. Seems interested in me.   (18)
    1   2   3   4   5

14. Has no time for me.   (19)
    1   2   3   4   5

15. Helps me to believe in myself.   (20)
    1   2   3   4   5

16. Keeps me informed.   (21)
    1   2   3   4   5

17. Fails to keep his/her promises to me.   (22)
    1   2   3   4   5

18. Encourages me to think for myself.   (23)
    1   2   3   4   5

19. Supports me with my beliefs.   (24)
    1   2   3   4   5

20. Encourages me to ask questions.   (25)
    1   2   3   4   5

21. Helps me see the positive aspects of my situation.   (26)
    1   2   3   4   5

22. Encourages me to continue working here.   (27)
    1   2   3   4   5

Since I have been a patient here, the nurses:

23. Anticipate my needs. (28)
    1   2   3   4   5

24. Encourages me to talk about my concerns. (29)
    1   2   3   4   5

25. Openly shows concern for me. (30)
    1   2   3   4   5

26. Asks me about my family. (31)
    1   2   3   4   5

27. Never shows any emotion. (32)
    1   2   3   4   5

28. Asks me how I would do things. (33)
    1   2   3   4   5

29. Helps me deal with any negative feelings. (34)
    1   2   3   4   5

30. Shares personal information with me when appropriate. (35)
    1   2   3   4   5

31. Expresses human emotions when he/she is with me. (36)
    1   2   3   4   5

32. Responds honestly to my questions. (37)
    1   2   3   4   5

33. Initiates conversations with me. (38)
    1   2   3   4   5

34. Checks on me frequently. (39)
    1   2   3   4   5

35. Looks me in the eye when he/she talks to me. (40)
    1   2   3   4   5

36. Refuses to tell me aspects about my work when I ask. (41)
    1   2   3   4   5

37. Pays attention to me when I am talking. (42)
    1   2   3   4   5

38. Acts as if he/she disapproves of me. (43)
    1   2   3   4   5

Since I have been a patient here, the nurses:

39. Encourages me to talk about whatever is on my mind.   (44)
    1   2   3   4   5

40. Is patient with me even when I am difficult.   (45)
    1   2   3   4   5

41. Is interested in information I have to offer.   (46)
    1   2   3   4   5

42. Talks about me openly in front of other staff.   (47)
    1   2   3   4   5

43. Accepts what I say, even if it is negative.   (48)
    1   2   3   4   5

44. Seems annoyed if I speak my true feelings.   (49)
    1   2   3   4   5

45. Is aware of my feelings.   (50)
    1   2   3   4   5

46. Does not want to talk to me.   (51)
    1   2   3   4   5

47. Allows me to talk about my true feelings without any risk to   (52)
    my position.
    1   2   3   4   5

48. Questions me about my past experiences in nursing.   (53)
    1   2   3   4   5

49. Helps me set career goals which I am able to accomplish. (54)
    1   2   3   4   5

50. Helps me find solutions regarding my problems.   (55)
    1   2   3   4   5

51. Deals with my work problems in ways that are impractical for   (56)
    me.
    1   2   3   4   5

52. Helps me with all my work problem/s, not just part of them.   (57)
    1   2   3   4   5

53. Helps me deal with difficult situations.   (58)
    1   2   3   4   5

Since I have been a patient here, the nurses:

54. Helps me understand my feelings. (59)
    1   2   3   4   5

55. Asks me how I think my work is going. (60)
    1   2   3   4   5

56. Helps me explore alternative ways of dealing with my work (61)
    problem/s.
    1   2   3   4   5

57. Provides me with literature regarding my work and areas of (62)
    interest.
    1   2   3   4   5

58. Uses management terms that I don't understand. (63)
    1   2   3   4   5

59. Knows what he/she is doing. (64)
    1   2   3   4   5

60. Teaches me about nursing and/or health care. (65)
    1   2   3   4   5

61. Discourages me from asking questions. (66)
    1   2   3   4   5

62. Checks with me to make sure I understand. (67)
    1   2   3   4   5

63. Makes me feel as comfortable as possible. (68)
    1   2   3   4   5

64. Tells me what to expect. (69)
    1   2   3   4   5

65. Knows when to go to a higher authority. (70)
    1   2   3   4   5

66. Respects my need for confidentiality. (71)
    1   2   3   4   5

67. Makes sure the charge nurse/assistant head nurse knows my (72)
    strengths and weaknesses.
    1   2   3   4   5

68. Knows what to do in an emergency. (73)
    1   2   3   4   5

Since I have been a patient here, the nurses:

69. Never asks what I need.   (74)
     1   2   3   4   5

70. Protects me from situations where I could get harmed.   (75)
     1   2   3   4   5

71. Knows a lot about my work habits.   (76)
     1   2   3   4   5

72. Spends time with me.   (77)
     1   2   3   4   5

73. Makes me feel secure regarding my position.   (78)
     1   2   3   4   5

74. Allows my family to call the unit.   (79)
     1   2   3   4   5

75. Limits or interferes with my routine practices.   (80)
     1   2   3   4   5

76. Makes sure I get to meals or have time out for my own needs.   (81)
     1   2   3   4   5

77. Monitors my skill level.   (82)
     1   2   3   4   5

78. Keeps me challenged.   (83)
     1   2   3   4   5

79. Makes sure my paycheck is accurate.   (84)
     1   2   3   4   5

80. Makes me wait a long time for an appointment when I need   (85)
     help.
     1   2   3   4   5

81. Helps me feel less worried.   (86)
     1   2   3   4   5

82. Allows me time off to be with my spouse and special family/   (87)
     friends.
     1   2   3   4   5

83. Discourages me from interacting with others.   (88)
     1   2   3   4   5

Since I have been a patient here, the nurses:

84. Helps me achieve my career goals. (89)
    1   2   3   4   5

85. Respects my needs when scheduling shifts. (90)
    1   2   3   4   5

86. Doesn't care whether I get a break. (91)
    1   2   3   4   5

87. Understands my unique situation. (92)
    1   2   3   4   5

88. Has no idea how this job is affecting my life. (93)
    1   2   3   4   5

89. Is concerned about how I view things. (94)
    1   2   3   4   5

90. Knows what is important to me. (95)
    1   2   3   4   5

91. Acknowledges my inner feelings. (96)
    1   2   3   4   5

92. Helps me cope with the stress of my work. (97)
    1   2   3   4   5

93. Shows respect for those things that have meaning for me. (98)
    1   2   3   4   5

94. Is out of touch with my daily world. (99)
    1   2   3   4   5

THIS IS THE END OF THE QUESTIONNAIRE. IF YOU WERE ASKED TO ADVISE HEAD NURSES/NURSE ADMINISTRATORS ON WHAT THEY NEED TO DO DIFFERENTLY, WHAT WOULD YOU ADVISE? YOU MAY WRITE ON THE BACK OF THIS PAGE. THANK YOU VERY MUCH FOR YOUR PARTICIPATION.

Code No. _____ (1–4)
Card No. _____ (5)

STUDENT NURSE SURVEY
CAT-EDU.*

Directions: All of the statements in this survey refer to activities that occur among people in a nursing school. There are five possible responses to each item. They are:

1 = Never
2 = Rarely
3 = Occasionally
4 = Frequently
5 = Always

For each statement, please circle how often you think each activity is occurring during your hospitalization.

Since I have been a student nurse here, my instructors:

1. Listen to me.   (6)
    1   2   3   4   5

2. Accept me as I am.   (7)
    1   2   3   4   5

3. Treat me kindly.   (8)
    1   2   3   4   5

4. Ignore me.   (9)
    1   2   3   4   5

5. Answer my questions.   (10)
    1   2   3   4   5

6. Include me in their discussions.   (11)
    1   2   3   4   5

---

*©Joanne R. Duffy, D.N.Sc., R.N., CCRN, 1990, Georgetown University School of Nursing, Washington, D.C.
Reprinted with permission of author.

Since I have been a patient here, the nurses:

7. Respect me. (12)
   1   2   3   4   5

8. Are more interested in their own problems. (13)
   1   2   3   4   5

9. Pay attention to me. (14)
   1   2   3   4   5

10. Enjoy working with me. (15)
    1   2   3   4   5

11. Use my name when they talk to me. (16)
    1   2   3   4   5

12. Are available to me. (17)
    1   2   3   4   5

13. Have no time for me. (18)
    1   2   3   4   5

14. Seem interested in me. (19)
    1   2   3   4   5

15. Support me with my beliefs. (20)
    1   2   3   4   5

16. Help me to believe my myself. (21)
    1   2   3   4   5

17. Keep me informed. (22)
    1   2   3   4   5

18. Fail to keep their promises to me. (23)
    1   2   3   4   5

19. Encourage me to think for myself. (24)
    1   2   3   4   5

20. Support me with my beliefs. (25)
    1   2   3   4   5

21. Encourage me to ask questions. (26)
    1   2   3   4   5

22. Help me see some good aspects of my situation. (27)
    1   2   3   4   5

Since I have been a patient here, the nurses:

23. Encourage me to continue studying here.   (28)
    1   2   3   4   5

24. Anticipate my needs.   (29)
    1   2   3   4   5

25. Encourage me to talk about my concerns.   (30)
    1   2   3   4   5

26. Openly show concern for me.   (31)
    1   2   3   4   5

27. Ask me about my family.   (32)
    1   2   3   4   5

28. Never show any emotion.   (33)
    1   2   3   4   5

29. Ask how I would do things.   (34)
    1   2   3   4   5

30. Help me deal with any negative feelings.   (35)
    1   2   3   4   5

31. When appropriate, share personal information with me.   (36)
    1   2   3   4   5

32. Express human emotions when they are with me.   (37)
    1   2   3   4   5

33. Respond honestly to my questions.   (38)
    1   2   3   4   5

34. Initiate conversations with me.   (39)
    1   2   3   4   5

35. Check on me frequently.   (40)
    1   2   3   4   5

36. Look me in the eye when they talk to me.   (41)
    1   2   3   4   5

37. Refuse to tell me aspects about my performance when I ask. (42)
    1   2   3   4   5

Since I have been a patient here, the nurses:

38. Pay attention to me when I am talking. (43)
    1   2   3   4   5

39. Act as if they disapprove of me. (44)
    1   2   3   4   5

40. Encourage me to talk about whatever is on my mind. (45)
    1   2   3   4   5

41. Are patient with me even when I am difficult. (46)
    1   2   3   4   5

42. Are interested in information I have to offer. (47)
    1   2   3   4   5

43. Talk about me openly in front of other faculty. (48)
    1   2   3   4   5

44. Accept what I say, even when it is negative. (49)
    1   2   3   4   5

45. Seem annoyed if I speak my true feelings. (50)
    1   2   3   4   5

46. Are aware of my feelings. (51)
    1   2   3   4   5

47. Don't want to talk to me. (52)
    1   2   3   4   5

48. Allow me to talk about my true feelings without any risk to (53)
    my grades.
    1   2   3   4   5

49. Question me about my past experiences in nursing. (54)
    1   2   3   4   5

50. Help me set career goals that I am able to accomplish. (55)
    1   2   3   4   5

51. Help me find solutions regarding my problems. (56)
    1   2   3   4   5

52. Deal with my school problems in ways that are impractical (57)
    for me.
    1   2   3   4   5

Since I have been a patient here, the nurses:

53. Help me with all of my school problems, not just part of   (58)
    them.
    1   2   3   4   5

54. Help me deal with difficult situations.   (59)
    1   2   3   4   5

55. Help me understand my feelings.   (60)
    1   2   3   4   5

56. Ask me how I think my school work is going.   (61)
    1   2   3   4   5

57. Help me explore alternative ways of dealing with my school   (62)
    problems.
    1   2   3   4   5

58. Know when to go to a higher authority.   (63)
    1   2   3   4   5

59. Provide me with literature regarding my work and areas of   (64)
    interest.
    1   2   3   4   5

60. Use terms I don't understand.   (65)
    1   2   3   4   5

61. Know what they are doing.   (66)
    1   2   3   4   5

62. Help me to learn about nursing and/or health care.   (67)
    1   2   3   4   5

63. Discourage me from asking questions.   (68)
    1   2   3   4   5

64. Check with me to make sure I understand.   (69)
    1   2   3   4   5

65. Tell me what to expect.   (70)
    1   2   3   4   5

66. Make me feel as comfortable as possible.   (71)
    1   2   3   4   5

67. Respect my need for confidentiality.   (72)
    1   2   3   4   5

Since I have been a patient here, the nurses:

68. Make sure that other instructors know my strengths and weak- (73)
nesses.
  1   2   3   4   5

69. Know what to do in an emergency. (74)
  1   2   3   4   5

70. Never ask what I need. (75)

  1   2   3   4   5

71. Protect me from situations where I could get harmed. (76)
  1   2   3   4   5

72. Know a lot about try work habits. (77)
  1   2   3   4   5

73. Spend time with me. (78)
  1   2   3   4   5

74. Make me feel secure regarding my performance in school. (79)
  1   2   3   4   5

75. Allow my family to make demands on me. (80)
  1   2   3   4   5

76. Limit or interfere with my basic routine practices. (81)
  1   2   3   4   5

77. Make sure I have time out for my own needs. (82)
  1   2   3   4   5

78. Keep me challenged. (83)
  1   2   3   4   5

79. Monitor my skill level. (84)
  1   2   3   4   5

80. Make sure my grades are accurate. (85)
  1   2   3   4   5

81. Make me wait a long time for an appointment when I need (86)
help.
  1   2   3   4   5

82. Help me feel less worried. (87)
  1   2   3   4   5

Since I have been a patient here, the nurses:

83. Allow me the time to be with my spouse and special family/   (88)
    friends.
    1   2   3   4   5

84. Discourage me from interacting with others.   (89)
    1   2   3   4   5

85. Help me achieve my career goals.   (90)
    1   2   3   4   5

86. Don't care whether I get a break.   (91)
    1   2   3   4   5

87. Respects my needs when scheduling class and/or clinicals.   (92)
    1   2   3   4   5

88. Understand my unique situation.   (93)
    1   2   3   4   5

89. Have no idea how school is affecting my life.   (94)
    1   2   3   4   5

90. Are concerned about how I view things.   (95)
    1   2   3   4   5

91. Know what is important to me.   (96)
    1   2   3   4   5

92. Acknowledge my inner feelings.   (97)
    1   2   3   4   5

93. Help me cope with the stress of my educational experiences.   (98)
    1   2   3   4   5

94. Show respect for those things that have meaning for me.   (99)
    1   2   3   4   5

95. Are out of touch with my daily world.   (100)
    1   2   3   4   5

THIS IS THE END OF THE QUESTIONNAIRE. IF YOU WERE ASKED TO ADVISE FACULTY ON WHAT THEY NEED TO DO DIFFERENTLY, WHAT WOULD YOU ADVISE? YOU MAY WRITE ON THE BACK OF THIS PAGE. THANK YOU VERY MUCH FOR YOUR PARTICIPATION.

13

Peer Group Caring Interaction Scale and Organizational Climate for Caring Questionnaire

(Hughes, 1998)

PEER GROUP CARING INTERACTION SCALE

The Peer Group Caring Interaction Scale (PGCIS) is a summated rating scale designed by Hughes (1993) to measure the climate for caring as experienced among a student peer group. The PGCIS is one of two investigator-developed instruments which focus on the climate for caring among students in nursing education. The second tool by Hughes, the Organizational Climate for Caring Questionnaire (OCCQ), will be addressed separately. The original PGCIS was empirically derived from data that were generated in a qualitative study conducted with ten junior nursing students enrolled in five BSN schools of nursing. There was no formally identified conceptual-theoretical basis for the instrument, except for general interest in identifying behavioral and interactional aspects of caring as experienced by nursing students. However, theories of caring and education are evident in the direction, nature, and application of the instrument. Caring curricular ideas and educational theories of caring, as described by Bevis (Bevis & Watson, 2000), along with Noddings (1984), are built into the assumptions upon which the original study was conducted. However, they were not explicitly identified as the theoretical-conceptual basis of the instrument development, but were noted in the general background of the original work.

The PGCIS was constructed to include two subscales: Modeling and Giving Assistance. The modeling subscale includes nine items that describe peer behaviors through which presence/willingness to help, sensitivity, and supportiveness are conveyed. The giving assistance subscale has seven items that describe actions perceived as caring by peers, such as sharing information, sharing ideas, and sharing aspects of the self.

The PGCIS was pretested for face validity with a convenience sample of 10 junior students, enrolled in a single baccalaureate nursing program. Content validity was based upon item review by two nurse educators with content expertise in the concept of caring. The revised PGCIS was pilot tested in a study with 873 nursing students in 87 schools of nursing, randomly selected from the *1992 Edition of State Approved Schools of Nursing.* Cronbach's alpha for each subscale was reported to be .91. The mean inter-item correlation for the two subscales was .60, suggesting minimum redundancy among items.

The final 16-item version of the PGCIS was subjected to exploratory factor analysis using maximum likelihood estimation. The proposed two-factor solution accounted for 59% of the total variance and adequately reproduced the observed correlations with no residuals exceeding .10. Thus, empirical support has been established for the two-factor structure of the instrument. PGCIS scores have been positively correlated with scores on the intimacy subscale of the OCDQ and the Peer Group Interaction Scale, and negatively correlated with scores on the disengagement subscale of the OCDQ (.59, .69, and .54, respectively, all at P < .001 levels). These correlations provide beginning support for PGCIS validity using the convergent and divergent validity approaches.

Hughes (2001) concludes that there is preliminary support for the PGCIS as a reliable and valid approach to the measurement of peer group caring in baccalaureate schools of nursing. She further suggests that the PGCIS has potential applicability in the evaluation of the "hidden" curriculum as described by Bevis (Bevis & Watson, 2000); thus it can be used to examine educational strategies designed to enhance students' caring interactions.

The Peer Group Caring Interaction Scale is one of the few caring measurements that are designed for use in nursing education, and is the only one in the project found to focus on peer group climate. This instrument is copyrighted and the author requests that she be contacted for additional information and permission for its use. The original work for this instrument's development was supported by the NIH, National Center for Nursing Research, Predoctoral Fellowship No.1 F31NR06531 and a summer research grant from Kansas Health Foundation. A matrix framework with key summary data for the PGCIS is included in the table which follows the discussion of Hughes' Scale: Organizational Climate for Caring Questionnaire (OCCQ).

ORGANIZATIONAL CLIMATE FOR CARING QUESTIONNAIRE (HUGHES, 1993, 2001)

The Organizational Climate for Caring Questionnaire (OCCQ) is a sister measurement tool to the PGCIS. It is a newly reported instrument and as of yet has not been published. This instrument was developed as part of the author's doctoral dissertation which was funded by NIH-NINR, Predoctoral Fellowship #1 F31 NR06531 (Hughes, 1993, 2001).

The OCCQ was constructed and refined over a series of three pilot studies designed to capture dimensions of a caring climate experienced by nursing students. The interest of the investigator was related to normative educational processes and the environmental contexts within which caring can be learned. The student perceived organizational climate for caring within the context of faculty-student interactions, was the focus for study and instrument construction. OCCQ items were based upon data obtained during individual interviews with ten junior students enrolled at five baccalaureate schools of nursing who were asked to describe a climate of caring within the context of their interactions with faculty.

The conceptual-theoretical basis of the instrument is Noddings' (1984) conceptualizations of the components of a moral education for a caring curriculum. The OCCQ consists of four subscales which correspond directly with Nodding's framework for caring in education: Modeling, Dialogue, Practice, and Confirmation. The modeling subscale has 14 items that describe caring behaviors that can be modeled by teachers during their interactions with students. The dialogue subscale has nine items that describe the open exchange of thoughts, ideas, or opinions between teachers and students. The practice subscale has nine items that focus on students' clinical practice experiences. The confirmation subscale has seven items that address the role of teachers in building students' self-esteem by expressing confidence in their ability and potential as students and future nurses.

Two content experts helped to establish the content validity of the OCCQ (Hughes, 1993, 2001). Three pilot studies to develop psychometric properties of the OCCQ were conducted with junior students enrolled at NLN-accredited baccalaureate schools of nursing randomly selected from state-approved schools of nursing. The samples included 180 students from 20 schools for Pilot # 1, 363 students from 27 schools for Pilot # 2, and 853 students from 87 schools for Pilot # 3.

Hughes used Pilot # 3 data to establish psychometric properties. Coefficient alphas for the OCCQ subscales ranged from .88 to .92. (Hughes, 2001). Convergent validity was assessed by correlating scores on the OCCQ and subscales on two other scales. Correlations ranged from .50 to .86. Separate factor analyses using maximum likelihood estimation were completed in Pilots # 2 and # 3 in which four factors resulted: Modeling/Dialogue, Practice, Confirmation, and Uncaring Behaviors.

Hughes (2001) reports that the combined findings of the studies on the OCCQ suggest that this instrument offers a reliable and valid approach to the measurement of the organizational climate for caring in schools of nursing. This concept is conceptualized as a variable that mediates the relationship between student outcomes and the educational process. Assessment of the organizational climate for caring within the context of faculty-student relationships can be useful in the evaluation of nursing education programs. The OCCQ is the only tool on caring identified for this project that specifically addresses organizational climate for caring in nursing education. While no published reports exist yet for the OCCQ, this tool has promise for future refinement, testing, and use in nursing educational research, both at the individual student perceptional level, as well as at the organizational climate level.

This instrument is copyrighted by Hughes (1993, 2001). The author requests that anyone wishing to use the OCCQ contact her for more information. Any published research using the instrument should indicate Hughes as the author of the instrument. Table 13.1 presents a matrix of key properties for both the PGCIS and the OCCQ instruments.

TABLE 13.1 Matrix of Peer Group Caring Interaction Scale (Hughes, 1993, 1998) and Organizational Climate for Caring Questionnaire (Hughes, 1993)

Instrument & Year Developed	Author and Contact Information	Publication Source Citation	Developed to Measure	Instrument Description	Participants	Reported Validity/ Reliability	Conceptual-Theoretical Basis of Measurement	Latest Citation in Nursing Literature
Peer Group Caring Interaction Scale (PGCIS) 1993, 1998	Linda Hughes Associate Professor Nursing, University of Texas Medical Branch, 301 University Blvd., Galveston, Texas 77555-1029 Ph: 409-772-8255 FAX 409 772 8323 *lchughes@ utmb.edu*	Hughes, L. (1993). Peer group interactions and the student perceived climate for caring. *Journal of Nursing Education, 32(2),* 78–83. Hughes, L. C. (1998). Development of an instrument to measure caring peer group interactions.	Organizational climate of caring perceived among nursing student peer group	16 items; 6-point Likert with 2 subscales: Modeling & Giving Assistance	n = 873 BSN students at 87 NLN accredited, State approved schools of nursing	Cronbach's alpha .91 for each subscale Factor analysis; convergent validity based on positive correlations with the intimacy subscale of the OCDQ and the Peer Group Interaction Scale; Divergent validity based on negative	No formal conceptual-theoretical framework identified; but indirectly informed by caring literature and caring theories as well as educational theories, e.g. Noddings (1984) and Bevis (Bevis &	Hughes, L. C., Kosowski, M. M, Grams, K. & Wilson, C. (1998). Caring interactions among nursing students: A descriptive comparison of two associate degree nursing programs. *Nursing Outlook, 4(4),* 176–181. (Development of instrument,

(continued)

TABLE 13.1 *(continued)*

Instrument & Year Developed	Author and Contact Information	Publication Source Citation	Developed to Measure	Instrument Description	Participants	Reported Validity/ Reliability	Conceptual-Theoretical Basis of Measurement	Latest Citation in Nursing Literature
		correlation with the *Journal of Nursing Education, 37*(5), 202–207.				disengagement subscale of the OCDQ (Hughes, 1998)	Watson, 1989, 2000)	funded by Kansas Health Foundation, Summer Research Award)
Organizational Climate for Caring Questionnaire (OCCQ) Hughes, 1993	Hughes, as above	Hughes, L. (1993). *Relationships among the organizational characteristics of baccalaureate schools of nursing and the student-perceived organizational climate for caring.* Unpublished	Designed to measure student-perceived organizational climate for caring within context of faculty-student interactions	39 items and four subscales: Modeling, Dialogue, Practice, and Confirmation	Junior students enrolled at an accredited BSN school of nursing; Pilot #1: n = 180 students from 20 nursing schools; Pilot #2: n = 363 students from 27 schools;	3 pilot studies; content validity; alpha subscales ranged from .88 to .92; Convergent validity established; Factor analysis yielding four factors: Modeling, dialogue, Practice,	Noddings' caring ethic and moral development for caring curriculum	Huber, D. I., Maas, M., McCloskey, J., Scherb, C. A., Goode, C. J. & Watson, C. (2000). Evaluating nursing administration instruments. *Journal of Nursing Administration, 30*(5), 251–272. Development

TABLE 13.1 *(continued)*

Instrument & Year Developed	Author and Contact Information	Publication Source Citation	Developed to Measure	Instrument Description	Participants	Reported Validity/ Reliability	Conceptual- Theoretical Basis of Measurement	Latest Citation in Nursing Literature
		Doctoral Dissertation. The University of Texas at Austin. Hughes, L. A (1992). Faculty-student interactions and the student-perceived climate for caring. *ANS*, *14*(3), 60–71.			Pilot #3: n = 853 students from 87 schools	Confirmation, Uncaring Behaviors		of instrument funded by NIH-NINR, Predoctoral Fellowship #1 F31 NR06531

157

PEER GROUP CARING INTERACTION SCALE*

Developed by
Linda C. Hughes, PhD, RN
Associate Professor, School of Nursing
University of Texas Medical Branch
301 University Blvd.
Galveston, TX 77555-1029
(409) 772-8247

Directions:
Please respond to each of the statements listed below by circling the number that best describes the climate or atmosphere at YOUR school of nursing. Make your responses according to how things are at your school *NOT* how you would like them to be or how you think they should be.

		Strongly Disagree	Moderately Disagree	Slightly Disagree	Slightly Agree	Moderately Agree	Strongly Agree
1.	Students at this school anticipate the needs of their classmates.	1	2	3	4	5	6
2.	Students at this school talk with each other about their problems and concerns.	1	2	3	4	5	6
3.	Students at this school share ideas with each other about how to best take care of patients.	1	2	3	4	5	6
4.	Students at this school talk to their classmates about things they wish they had done better while in a patient care setting.	1	2	3	4	5	6

*Reprinted by permission of author.
©Copyright L. Hughes.

	Strongly Disagree	Moderately Disagree	Slightly Disagree	Slightly Agree	Moderately Agree	Strongly Agree
5. Students at this school will help a classmate ONLY WHEN it is in their best interest to do so.	1	2	3	4	5	6
6. Students at this school think it should be left up to the teachers to work with students who need extra help.	1	2	3	4	5	6
7. There is a lot of camaraderie among the students at this school.	1	2	3	4	5	6
8. Students at this school notice when a classmate is having problems.	1	2	3	4	5	6
9. Students at this school get advice and suggestions from their classmates when completing homework assignments.	1	2	3	4	5	6
10. Students at this school can count on their classmates for help.	1	2	3	4	5	6
11. Students at this school are TOO BUSY to help their classmates.	1	2	3	4	5	6
12. Students at this school are a source of encouragement to each other.	1	2	3	4	5	6

		Strongly Disagree	Moderately Disagree	Slightly Disagree	Slightly Agree	Moderately Agree	Strongly Agree
13.	Students at this school help each other by sharing class notes, books, or articles.	1	2	3	4	5	6
14.	Students at this school get opinions from their classmates about things that happen to them while in a patient care setting.	1	2	3	4	5	6
15.	Students at this school talk with their classmates about how it feels to care for patients they are uncomfortable with.	1	2	3	4	5	6
16.	There is TOO MUCH competition among the students at this school.	1	2	3	4	5	6

Modeling Subscale:
Items 1, 5*, 6*, 7, 8, 10, 11*, 12, 16*

Giving Assistance Subscale:
Items 2, 3, 4, 9, 13, 14, 15

*Reverse Scored Items

ORGANIZATIONAL CLIMATE FOR CARING
QUESTIONNAIRE*

Developed by Linda Hughes, PhD, RN
Associate Professor, School of Nursing
University of Texas Medical Branch
301 University Blvd.
Galveston, TX 77555-1029
(409) 772-8247

DIRECTIONS:
Please respond to each of the statements listed below by circling the number that best describes the climate or atmosphere at YOUR school of nursing. Make your responses according to how things are at your school *NOT* how you would like things to be.

		Strongly Disagree	Moderately Disagree	Slightly Disagree	Slightly Agree	Moderately Agree	Strongly Agree
1.	The teachers at this school are always cheering the students on.	1	2	3	4	5	6
2.	Students at this school are given the reason for decisions that affect them.	1	2	3	4	5	6
3.	There is an open exchange of ideas among teachers and students at this school.	1	2	3	4	5	6
4.	Students at this school get a lot of uplifting encouragement from the teachers.	1	2	3	4	5	6
5.	The teachers at this school sincerely want to see students succeed.	1	2	3	4	5	6

*Reprinted by permission of author.

	Strongly Disagree	Moderately Disagree	Slightly Disagree	Slightly Agree	Moderately Agree	Strongly Agree
6. The teachers at this school are easy to talk to.	1	2	3	4	5	6
7. The teachers at this school tell students up front what is expected of them.	1	2	3	4	5	6
8. The teachers at this school DO NOT make students feel stupid for asking questions.	1	2	3	4	5	6
9. The teachers at this school help students have confidence in themselves.	1	2	3	4	5	6
10. The teachers at this school take a personal interest in students.	1	2	3	4	5	6
11. Students at this school can depend on the clinical teachers to help them do a good job of taking care of patients.	1	2	3	4	5	6
12. Students at this school can count on a pat on the back from their teachers when they perform well.	1	2	3	4	5	6
13. Students at this school can NEVER be sure how the teachers will treat them from one day to the next.	1	2	3	4	5	6

	Strongly Disagree	Moderately Disagree	Slightly Disagree	Slightly Agree	Moderately Agree	Strongly Agree
14. The clinical teachers at this school sometimes put students down in front of other people.	1	2	3	4	5	6
15. The teachers at this school understand how it feels to be a student.	1	2	3	4	5	6
16. The teachers at this school take the time to make sure that students understand what they are learning.	1	2	3	4	5	6
17. The teachers at this school make it a point to tell students that they have confidence in their ability to become good nurses.	1	2	3	4	5	6
18. Conflicts between teachers and students at this school can be resolved through one-to-one meetings.	1	2	3	4	5	6
19. The teachers at this school tell students what they are doing wrong RATHER THAN what they are doing right.	1	2	3	4	5	6
20. At this school, it is very much "I'm the instructor and you're the student and this is how we do it."	1	2	3	4	5	6

		Strongly Disagree	Moderately Disagree	Slightly Disagree	Slightly Agree	Moderately Agree	Strongly Agree
21.	The teachers at this school recognize when students are having problems.	1	2	3	4	5	6
22.	The clinical teachers at this school make it possible for students to do their best when taking care of patients.	1	2	3	4	5	6
23.	The teachers at this school enjoy being around students.	1	2	3	4	5	6
24.	The teachers at this school are usually TOO BUSY to take time to really listen to students' problems or concerns.	1	2	3	4	5	6
25.	The teachers at this school deal with students fairly.	1	2	3	4	5	6
26.	Students and teachers at this school share personal experiences with each other.	1	2	3	4	5	6
27.	Students at this school think it is a WASTE OF TIME to talk with the teachers about their problems.	1	2	3	4	5	6
28.	The teachers at this school take students' opinions into account when deciding about school policies and procedures.	1	2	3	4	5	6

		Strongly Disagree	Moderately Disagree	Slightly Disagree	Slightly Agree	Moderately Agree	Strongly Agree
29.	The clinical teachers at this school ADD to the anxiety that students feel in the clinical setting.	1	2	3	4	5	6
30.	The clinical teachers at this school give more attention to evaluating students than to helping students meet patients' needs.	1	2	3	4	5	6
31.	Students at this school feel free to state their ideas or opinions around the teachers.	1	2	3	4	5	6
32.	The clinical teachers at this school help students problem-solve difficult patient situations.	1	2	3	4	5	6
33.	It is safe for students at this school to openly disagree with the teachers.	1	2	3	4	5	6
34.	The teachers at this school treat each student as an individual.	1	2	3	4	5	6
35.	The clinical teachers at this school set a good example for students in their behaviors with patients and families.	1	2	3	4	5	6

	Strongly Disagree	Moderately Disagree	Slightly Disagree	Slightly Agree	Moderately Agree	Strongly Agree
36. The clinical teachers at this school are genuinely concerned about the patients to whom the students are assigned.	1	2	3	4	5	6
37. As nurses, the teachers at this school know what they are doing.	1	2	3	4	5	6
38. The teachers at this school are readily available to students.	1	2	3	4	5	6
39. The clinical teachers at this school make it easy for students to perform well in the clinical setting.	1	2	3	4	5	6

14

Caring Efficacy Scale

(Coates, 1995, 1997)

The Caring Efficacy Scale (CES) was developed by Dr. Carolie Coates, currently a consultant in the area of measurement and program evaluation. It was designed to assess one's confidence (or sense of efficacy) about one's ability to express a caring orientation, and establish a caring relationship, with patients. The conceptual-theoretical basis for the scale is Bandura's Self-Efficacy Theory from the discipline of social psychology, and Watson's Theory of Transpersonal Human Caring, from nursing. The orientation for the most current version of the instrument, aside from the theories, is to evaluate outcomes of nursing education in a new, advanced program with a formal caring philosophy and caring curriculum (Watson & Phillips, 1992). The original CES self-report scale was adapted so it could be administered to nursing students, clinical preceptors, supervisors, alumni, and alumni employers to assess caring efficacy as an outcome of nursing curriculum at the University of Colorado School of Nursing.

The original version of the CES, drafted in the late 1980s and refined for application in 1992, had 46 items that attempted to measure caring attitudes, skills, and behaviors on a 6-point Likert scale, with a self-report format. Since then the CES has undergone a series of additional testing and revisions, resulting in the current 30-item, self-report scale and a parallel 30-item form designed for use by nurse preceptors/supervisors to rate a particular nurse. The current CES form is balanced for number of positive and negative items. For accreditation assessment, the two "long" forms for self-report and supervisors cited above were reduced to 12-item "short" versions on the basis of selecting the top 12 loading items in a factor analysis (Coates, 1997).

The initial version was tested on a sample of 47 novice nurses; this study produced promising reliability and validity information and provided guidance for reduction of items based on inter-item correlation. Later samples included 110 graduating nurses (BS, ND, and MS), 119 alumni (BS, ND, and MS), 117 employers of alumni, and 67 clinical preceptors supervising BS, ND, and MS nursing students. Nursing educational evaluation studies which used both the long and short forms of the CES produced good scale reliability data. Form A with 30 items (scale unbalanced with more positive than negative items) yielded an alpha of .85 and Form B with 30 items/current version (balanced for positively and negatively worded items) yielded an alpha .88. The alpha for the short form (12 items) of the supervisor scale was .84.

Content validity was established by having faculty members very familiar with Watson's Theory rate each of 30 items in Form B in terms of Watson's Carative Factors (Coates, 1997). A factor analysis conducted on the short form produced a three-factor solution accounting for 69% of the variance (Coates, 1996, unpublished). Items loading on Factor 1 (accounting for 41% of the variance) referred to sense of efficacy in establishing caring relationships with clients.

Additional concurrent validity evidence was provided by assessing the degree of relationship between the CES as a measure of caring, and the Clinical Evaluation Tool (CET) used by the University in accreditation studies as a measure of clinical competence. The CET achieved alphas of .85 for student self-ratings and .95 for supervisor ratings of students. Positive correlations were found between graduates' rating of care (CES) and their clinical competence ratings: Form A: $r = .34$ (p = .05); Form B: $r = .37$ (p = .01). Similar results occurred with alumni responses: $r = .63$ (p = .01). More important, alumni self-ratings on the CET correlated positively with the independent ratings employers made on the CET, $r = .46$ (p = .01).

In a more recent unpublished application (Coates, 1999) to assess the effects of a three-day training based on empowerment and Watson's Caring Theory, the CES achieved alphas of .91 on the pre-test utilization of the scale and .84 on the post-test. The sample was 118 health care workers in a rehabilitation hospital. Significant positive short-term change (post-test within 4–6 weeks) was established using the CES (p = .000). The CES correlated in predictable ways with other outcome measures; it correlated positively with personal accomplishment (Maslach Burnout Inventory), and negatively with reliance on powerful others, reliance on chance, depersonalization, and the job stress inventory. This additional research adds further credibility to the use of the tool in both clinical settings and educational program evaluation.

This tool is guided by theories from both social psychology and nursing caring theory. It has been tested in nursing education and clinical care settings. It has psychometric sophistication in its development, use, and refinement. The Likert form makes it relatively easy to use. It is one of the few caring measurement tools that offers content validity with reference to carative factors in Watson's theory. Coates reports that many schools of nursing in the U.S. have requested permission to use the CES as a student outcome measure. Since it is a copyrighted instrument the author requests that you contact her for permission to use it. A matrix of the Caring Efficacy Scale with overall summary information is included in Table 14.1 below.

TABLE 14.1 Matrix of Caring Efficacy Scale (Coates, 1995, 1997)

Instrument & Year Developed	Author & Contact Address	Year Publication Source Citation	Developed to Measure	Instrument Description	Participants	Reported Reliability/Validity	Conceptual-Theoretical Basis of Measurement	Latest Citation in Nursing Literature
Caring Efficacy Scale 1992, 1995	Carolie Coates, PhD Research & Measurement Consultant, 1441 Snowmass Ct., Boulder, Colorado 80303 303-499-5756 Coatescj@home.com	Coates, C. (1997). The Caring Efficacy Scale: Nurses' self-reports of caring in practice settings. *Advanced Practice Nursing Quarterly*, 3(1), 53–59.	Assess conviction or belief in one's ability to express a caring orientation, develop caring relationship with patients	Original 46 items 6-point Likert-type scale Current has 30 items (both self-report and supervisor format) Short Form 12 items	n = 110 nursing students n = 119 alumni n = 117 alumni employers n = 67 clinical supervisors	Cronbach's alpha Form A = .85; Form B = .88; shorter version of Form B = .84 Content validity against Theory/Watson's Carative factors Significant positive correlation between Clinical Evaluation Tool (alpha .85 and .95) and CES	Bandura's social psychology Self-Efficacy Scale and Watson's Caring Theory/10 Carative factors	Coates, C. (1997). The Caring Efficacy Scale: Nurses' self-reports of caring in practice settings. *Advanced Practice Nursing Quarterly*, 3(1), 53–59.

CARING EFFICACY SCALE*

Reprinted by permission of author
Coates, 1995, 1997

Instructions: When you are completing these items, think of your recent work with patients/clients in clinical settings. Circle the number that best expresses your opinion.

Rating Scale:

−3	strongly disagree	+1	slightly agree
−2	moderately disagree	+2	moderately agree
−1	slightly disagree	+3	strongly agree

		strongly disagree				strongly agree	
1.	I do not feel confident in my ability to express a sense of caring to my clients/patients.	−3	−2	−1	+1	+2	+3
2.	If I am not relating well to a client/patient, I try to analyze what I can do to reach him/her.	−3	−2	−1	+1	+2	+3
3.	I feel comfortable in touching my clients/patients in the course of caregiving.	−3	−2	−1	+1	+2	+3
4.	I convey a sense of personal strength to my clients/patients.	−3	−2	−1	+1	+2	+3
5.	Clien ts/patients can tell me most anything and I won't be shocked.	−3	−2	−1	+1	+2	+3
6.	I have an ability to introduce a sense of normalcy in stressful conditions.	−3	−2	−1	+1	+2	+3
7.	It is easy for me to consider the multifacets of a client's/patient's care, at the same time as I am listening to them.	−3	−2	−1	+1	+2	+3
8.	I have difficulty in suspending my personal beliefs and biases in order to hear and accept a client/patient as a person.	−3	−2	−1	+1	+2	+3
9.	I can walk into a room with a presence of serenity and energy that makes clients/patients feel better.	−3	−2	−1	+1	+2	+3

---

*©Carolie J. Coates. Reprinted by permission of author.

		strongly disagree				strongly agree	
10.	I am able to tune into a particular client/patient and forget my personal concerns.	−3	−2	−1	+1	+2	+3
11.	I can usually create some way to relate to most any client/patient.	−3	−2	−1	+1	+2	+3
12.	I lack confidence in my ability to talk to clients/patients from backgrounds different from my own.	−3	−2	−1	+1	+2	+3
13.	I feel if I talk to clients/patients on an individual, personal basis, things might get out of control.	−3	−2	−1	+1	+2	+3
14.	I use what I learn in conversations with clients/patients to provide more individualized care.	−3	−2	−1	+1	+2	+3
15.	I don't feel strong enough to listen to the fears and concerns of my clients/patients.	−3	−2	−1	+1	+2	+3
16.	Even when I'm feeling self-confident about most things, I still seem to be unable to relate to clients/patients.	−3	−2	−1	+1	+2	+3
17.	I seem to have trouble relating to clients/patients.	−3	−2	−1	+1	+2	+3
18.	I can usually establish a close relationship with my clients/patients.	−3	−2	−1	+1	+2	+3
19.	I can usually get patients/clients to like me.	−3	−2	−1	+1	+2	+3
20.	I often find it hard to get my point of view across to patients/clients when I need to.	−3	−2	−1	+1	+2	+3
21.	When trying to resolve a conflict with a client/patient, I usually make it worse.	−3	−2	−1	+1	+2	+3
22.	If I think a client/patient is uneasy or may need some help, I approach that person.	−3	−2	−1	+1	+2	+3
23.	If I find it hard to relate to a client/patient, I'll stop trying to work with that person.	−3	−2	−1	+1	+2	+3
24.	I often find it hard to relate to clients/patients from a different culture than mine.	−3	−2	−1	+1	+2	+3

		strongly disagree				strongly agree	
25.	I have helped many clients/patients through my ability to develop close, meaningful relationships.	−3	−2	−1	+1	+2	+3
26.	I often find it difficult to express empathy with clients/patients.	−3	−2	−1	+1	+2	+3
27.	I often become overwhelmed by the nature of the problems clients/patients are experiencing.	−3	−2	−1	+1	+2	+3
28.	When a client/patient is having difficulty communicating with me, I am able to adjust to his/her level.	−3	−2	−1	+1	+2	+3
29.	Even when I really try, I can't get through to difficult clients/patients.	−3	−2	−1	+1	+2	+3
30.	I don't use creative or unusual ways to express caring to my clients/patients.	−3	−2	−1	+1	+2	+3

© The Caring Efficacy Scale (CES) is copyrighted. This is the 30-item self-report form. Please contact Carolie J. Coates, Ph.D., Research and Measurement Consultant, 1441 Snowmass Court, Boulder, Colorado 80305, U.S.A., to formally request to use the Caring Efficacy Scale (CES). (An administrator/supervisor version (30-items) is also available, as well as short forms (12-items) of the self-report and administrator/supervisor version.)
Telephone and Fax +(303) 499-5756
E-mail: *coatescj@home.com*
(1/9/2001)

15

Holistic Caring Inventory

(Latham, 1988, 1996)

The Holistic Caring Inventory (HCI) was developed by Latham (1988, 1996) as part of her doctoral studies. The conceptual-theoretical basis of the instrument is Howard's (1975) holistic dimensions of humanistic caring theory. The most recent description of the instrument is in Latham (1996) in which the tool was used in a study examining predictors of patient outcomes following (caring) interactions with nurses.

The HCI is constructed as a four-point summated Likert scale; each item is rated on a continuum of (1) strongly disagree to (4) strongly agree. A mean score of 1 indicates that caring was not perceived, 2 means that some caring was evident, and scores 3 to 4 reflect moderate to high levels of caring (Latham, 1996). The instrument has a total of 39 items, comprising 4 subscales, i.e., Physical, Interpretive, Spiritual, and Sensitive.

Content validity was established by two caring experts, and discriminant validity was reportedly established with Kiesler's (1987) Impact Message Inventory in a study of 218 hospitalized patients. In the 1996 study by Latham, Cronbach alpha's for the four caring subscales were .89 (Interpretative) to .91 (Spiritual) with the other two (Physical and Sensitive) at .90. This instrument would be considered a first generation tool to measure caring, but has been refined and retested with additional research since its early development in 1988. Latham reports that continued refinement of caring concepts, with an emphasis on considering various levels of professional involvement is still needed. There is limited information about the HCI found in the nursing literature. The 1996 citation and the proceedings of a measurement conference in 1988, both in publications by Latham, are the primary sources of information other than direct contact with the author. The instrument is copyrighted and anyone wishing to use it is requested to contact the author for additional information and updates. The matrix in Table 15.1 below summarizes the data to date that are available about the HCI.

TABLE 15.1   Matrix of Holistic Caring Inventory (Latham, 1988, 1996)

Instrument and Year	Author and Contact Address	Publication Source Citation	Developed to Measure	Instrument Description	Participants	Reported Validity/ Reliability	Conceptual-Theoretical Basis of Measurement	Latest Citation in Nursing Literature
Holistic Caring Inventory, Latham, 1988, 1996	Christine Pollack Latham, DNSc., RN, Professor & Dept. Chair, Nursing Department California State University, Fullerton, PO Box 6868, Fullerton, CA 92834-6868 FAX: 714 278 3338 Ph: 714 278 2291 Email: *clatham @fullerton.edu*	Latham, C. P. (1996). Predictors of patient outcomes following interactions with nurses. *Western Journal of Nursing Research, 18*(5), 548–564.	Humanistic caring; patients' perceptions of caring	39-item, Likert-type scale; four-point summation instrument, with 4 caring subscales: physical; interpretive, spiritual, & sensitive	1988 dev. and testing: n = 218 hospitalized patients; 1996: n = 120 acutely ill, hospitalized adults, from 2 medical units of 2 medical centers	Content validity via 2 caring experts; Discriminant validity reported; Cronbach's alpha for 4 subscales: Physical = .90; Interpretive = .89; Spiritual = .91; Sensitive = .90	Psychology theory: Howard (1975) Holistic Dimension of Humanistic Caring Theory	Latham, C. P. (1996). Predictors of patient outcomes following interactions with nurses. *Western Journal of Nursing Research, 18*(5), 548–564. Williams, S. A. (1998). Quality and care: patients' perceptions. *Journal Nursing Care Quality, 12*(6), 18–25.

HOLISTIC CARING INVENTORY*
LATHAM (1988)

GENERAL DIRECTIONS: For the remaining questions think of one particular registered nurse who had the greatest effect on you during your hospitalization.

Example: The following statement is an example of how to answer this survey:

	1 Strongly Disagree	2 Disagree	3 Agree	4 Strongly Agree
I am able to get information from nurses to help me deal with my condition		X		

This answer indicates that the person did not always get information from the registered nurse about his or her condition

Instructions: Place a check mark in the appropriate box to the right of each statement. Keep a specific registered nurse in mind who has taken care of you during your current hospitalization.

The following 10 statements refer to getting physical help from a nurse

	1 Strongly Disagree	2 Disagree	3 Agree	4 Strongly Agree
1. I am able to discuss my physical problems with the nurse.				
2. The nurse is sensitive to the possible effect that information may have on my recovery.				
3. The information given by the nurse about my physical problems helps me to adjust to my condition.				

---

*Reprinted by permission of author.
©Copyright Latham.

	1 Strongly Disagree	2 Disagree	3 Agree	4 Strongly Agree
4. The nurse considers my feelings when giving me information about my physical condition.				
5. The nurse shows concern about how my physical condition will affect other areas of my life.				
6. The nurse allows time for me to think over my physical problems.				
7. The nurse shares his/her view of my physical condition with me.				
8. The nurse helps me with my feelings about changes happening to my body.				
9. The nurse understands my condition, and this helps me to deal with physical problems.				
10. The nurse knows when I need help in dealing with physical problems.				

The following 10 statements refer to the way the nurse deals with your feelings:

	1 Strongly Disagree	2 Disagree	3 Agree	4 Strongly Agree
11. When I am depressed, the nurse leaves me alone.				
12. The nurse listens to my feelings when taking care of me.				
13. The nurse helps me to interpret the meaning of my feelings.				

	1 Strongly Disagree	2 Disagree	3 Agree	4 Strongly Agree

14. The nurse shares her/his feelings about my situation to help me understand my condition.
15. The nurse helps me to discuss my feelings when I need to make changes.
16. The nurse is sensitive to my feelings when I am trying to understand my condition.
17. The nurse shows concern for my feelings.
18. The nurse openly discusses my feelings to help me to adjust to being ill.
19. The nurse tells me how he/she sees my feelings affecting others who are close to me.
20. The nurse reacts to my feelings in a way that helps me to adjust to a new situation.

The following 10 statements refer to how nurses handle other important areas of your life:

	1 Strongly Disagree	2 Disagree	3 Agree	4 Strongly Agree

21. The nurse gives information about how my condition will affect other areas of my life.
22. The nurse allows me time to reflect on how my condition will affect my family, friends, etc.
23. The nurse talks about my condition to family, friends, or other people I go to for help.

	1 Strongly Disagree	2 Disagree	3 Agree	4 Strongly Agree
24. When I have a new condition, I find that the nurse is easy to talk to.				
25. The nurse helps me with feelings about my relationships with others.				
26. The nurse discusses how my condition will affect the sexual aspects of my life.				
27. The nurse shows concern about how my condition will affect the work or job that I am normally involved with.				
28. The nurse shares her/his view of how my family or friends are reacting to my situation.				
29. I find the nurse is interested in knowing what I have done, or would like to do, during my lifetime.				
30. The nurse is aware of my idiosyncrasies and other things important to my care.				

The following 10 statements refer to how the nurse handles your need for hope and spiritual needs.

	1 Strongly Disagree	2 Disagree	3 Agree	4 Strongly Agree
31. While ill, I feel the nurse had shown concern for my spiritual needs.				
32. The nurse considers my need for some hope when telling me about my condition.				
33. I find that the nurse encourages me to reflect on my spiritual needs.				

	1 Strongly Disagree	2 Disagree	3 Agree	4 Strongly Agree
34. The nurse recognizes that my spiritual beliefs may help me to adjust to new situations in my life.				
35. The nurse openly discusses how this situation fits into the rest of my life.				
36. The nurse helps me obtain spiritual guidance when I can't deal with difficult feelings.				
37. The nurse accepts my need to sometimes feel like the situation is out of my hands.				
38. The nurse is able to sense times when I need help from a higher power.				
39. The nurse assists me in obtaining religious or spiritual advice to help me deal with health-related situations.				
40. The nurse does *not* get involved with my spiritual needs.				

16

Caring Dimensions Inventory

(Watson & Lea, 1997)

The Caring Dimensions Inventory (CDI) was developed at the University of Edinburgh, Scotland to create a reliable quantitative tool to measure caring. The conceptual-theoretical basis for the tool was guided by an empirical approach to caring rather than a theoretical one, while acknowledging some of the general caring theory literature. The theoretical approaches sought were those that supported the operationalization of caring through specific taxonomies and measurements.

Some of the Major Caring Taxonomic Constructs (MTCC) of Leininger (1981) were identified as helpful notions, along with the Nursing Intervention Lexicon and Taxonomy (NILT) of Grobe & Hughes (1993). In addition to reviewing academic literature, a grounded critique was made of "popular" articles in United Kingdom nursing journal/newspapers to detect how the concept of caring was presented to the readership of such publications. Any articles that used the key word, "care" or "caring," between 1983 and 1993 in the *British Journal of Nursing, Nursing Times, The Nursing Standard,* and *Professional Nursing* were gleaned for the meaning of the concept. From 63 articles reviewed and retrieved through a computerized system, 14 themes emerged. The most common were: nurse-patient relationship (36 articles); nursing interventions (17 articles); nursing attitudes (16 articles); nursing skills (15 articles); and communication (16 articles) (Watson & Lea, 1997). In formalizing the development of the CDI, "general categories of care" (GCC) were developed from the review described above; the four most popular themes were used to classify the CDI questions in that they were believed to describe GCC. A total of 25 core items were included on the CDI.

The CDI questionnaire was administered to nurses and student nurses in a local health trust and to a student sample in a neighboring health trust between August 1994 and January 1995. A total of 1452 were returned, from a distribution of 3024, representing a 47% rate of return. Cronbach's alpha was used to establish reliability/internal consistency of the 25 core items at a .91 level. Additional construct analysis was conducted to determine if there was a significant relationship between age, sex, and CDI. Sophisticated analysis through use of Mokken scale and SPSS-PC+, along with a Spearman's correlation of age and a Kruskal-Wallis 1-way ANOVA of DCI Mokken scale scores for male and female subjects were all carried out, yielding a statistically significant result (at $P < 0.05$) suggesting a relationship between age and CDI Mokken scale score and differences between male and females. An interesting finding was that older nurses perceive more technical aspects of nursing work as being caring, in addition to psychosocial aspects. Males tend to perceive of nursing (caring) in more psychosocial terms than females (Watson & Lea, 1997).

With respect to content validity, it was demonstrated through the content findings of previous quantitative research on caring, as well as presentation of caring in popular nursing journals. Research of this instrument continues at the University of Hull, under the leadership of Roger Watson, with continuing involvement from Lea, now in Vancouver, British Columbia under the name Dr. Amandah Hoogbruin (2000). Factor analysis has demonstrated a four-factor structure (Lea et al., 1998) and the CDI has been used in one longitudinal study of student nurses in Scotland (Watson et al., 1999) and by Walsh (1999) in a study of nurse practitioners in England. The authors hold copyright to the instrument and they request anyone using the tool to contact them for permission. The matrix in Table 16.1 outlines the key elements of the CDI along with the latest citations of the work, referred to as the Edinburgh Caring Dimensions Inventory (1998).

TABLE 16.1   Matrix of Caring Dimensions Inventory (Watson & Lea, 1997)

Instrument and Year Developed	Author Contact Address	Year Publication & Source Citation	Developed to Measure	Instrument Description	Participants	Reported Reliability/ Validity	Conceptual-Theoretical Basis of Measurement	Latest Citation in Nursing Literature
Caring Dimensions Inventory (CDI) Watson & Lea, 1997	Roger Watson, PhD, Professor, Department of Nursing, The University of Hull, Cottingham Road, Hull, England HU6 7RX Dr. Amandah (Lea) Hoogbruin, PhD, Nursing Faculty, Kwantlen	Watson, R., Lea, A. (1997). The caring dimensions inventory (CDI): Content validity, reliability and scaling. *Journal of Advanced Nursing, 25,* 87–94.	Perceptions of caring from large sample of nurses	5-point Likert Scale with 41 questions: 25 core questions re: perceptions of caring	n = 1452 Nurses and nursing students	Cronbach's alpha = .91 Mokken Scaling and Spearman's correlation of age; Kruskal-Wallis 1-way ANOVA for male vs. female (p < 0.05) for age and sex differences in perceptions of caring	Empirical approach vs. theoretical basis, although caring theory that supported operationalizing of caring was influential	Lea, A, Watson, R., Deary, I. J. (1998). Caring in Nursing: A Multivariate Analysis. *Journal of Advanced Nursing, 28*(3), 662–671. Lea, A. & Watson, R. (1999). Research in

TABLE 16.1 *(continued)*

Instrument and Year Developed	Author Contact Address	Year Publication & Source Citation	Developed to Measure	Instrument Description	Participants	Reported Reliability/Validity	Conceptual-Theoretical Basis of Measurement	Latest Citation in Nursing Literature
	University College, 12666-72nd Avenue, Surrey, BC, CANADA V3W 2M8 *amandah@ interchange. ubc.ca*							brief. Perceptions of caring among nurses: the relationship to clinical area. *Journal of Clinical Nursing,* 8(5), 617–618. Walsh, M. (1999). Nurses and nurse practitioners 1: priorities in care. *Nursing Standard, 13*(24), 38–42.

(continued)

185

TABLE 16.1 (*continued*)

Instrument and Year Developed	Author Contact Address	Year Publication & Source Citation	Developed to Measure	Instrument Description	Participants	Reported Reliability/ Validity	Conceptual- Theoretical Basis of Measurement	Latest Citation in Nursing Literature
								Watson, R., Deary, I. J. & Lea, A. (1999). A longitudinal study into the perceptions of caring among nursing students using multivariate analysis of the Caring Dimension Inventory. *Journal of Advanced Nursing, 30,* 1080–1089.

CARING DIMENSIONS INVENTORY (CDI)*

Stem Question: "Do you consider the following aspects of nursing practice to be caring?"

Response on five-point Likert scale: 1 (strongly disagree) to 5 (strongly agree)

1. Assisting a patient with an activity of daily living (washing, dressing, etc.)
2. Making a pursing record about the patient
3. Feeling sorry for a patient
4. Getting to know the patient as a person
5. Explaining a clinical procedure to a patient
6. Being neatly dressed when working with a patient
7. Sitting with a patient
8. Exploring a patient's lifestyle
9. Reporting a patient's condition to a senior nurse
10. Being with a patient during a clinical procedure
11. Being honest with a patient
12. Organizing the work of others for a patient
13. Listening to a patient
14. Consulting with the doctor about a patient
15. Instructing a patient about an aspect of self-care (washing, dressing, etc.)
16. Sharing your personal problems with a patient
17. Keeping relatives informed about a patient
18. Measuring the vital signs of a patient (e.g., pulse and blood pressure)
19. Putting the needs of a patient before your own
20. Being technically competent with a clinical procedure
21. Involving a patient with his or her care
22. Giving reassurance about a clinical procedure
23. Providing privacy for a patient
24. Being cheerful with a patient
25. Observing the effects of a medication on a patient

---

*Reprinted by permission of the authors.
©Copyright Watson & Lea.

17

Caring Attributes, Professional Self-Concept Technological Influences Scale

(Arthur et al., 1998, 1999)

Arthur and colleagues in Hong Kong (Arthur et al., 1998) developed a complex caring instrument and tested it with 1,957 registered nurses in 11 different countries. The purpose was to develop an understanding of caring, and to compare the responses of caring items with items related to professional self-concept and technological influences across diverse countries and cultures. The conceptual-theoretical basis of the study was informed by the earlier empirical work of Lea and Watson (Watson & Lea, 1996, 1997) and the conceptual and multidimensional construct development of Wolf et al. (1994). In addition, theoretical, practical, and pedagogical perspectives were generated from the general nursing caring literature, citing such works as Leininger (1981), Benner (1988), and Watson (1988), among others.

The early development of the Caring Attributes, Professional Self-Concept Technological Influences Scale (CAPSTI) was conducted through a pilot study, using a convenience sample of nurses from Hong Kong, Beijing, and Macau. The themes and language which emerged from this sample were reviewed for content validity by a sample of experts. The selection of specific items emerged from a combination of sources; the literature, the sample, and the experts. An additional sample of 100 nurses in Hong Kong were administered the instrument for establishing reliability and validity. Internal consistency was found to be greater than Cronbach's alpha of .7 for each part (Arthur et al., 1999). The four parts include 7 demographic items in part one; 30 items in the Professional Self-Concept of Nurses Instrument (PSCNI) in part two; part three includes technological influences (14 items); part four has 60 items related to caring.

The actual testing of the instrument consisted of Likert scales within the four parts identified. The high score corresponds with a positive attitude or belief. Individual scores and group scores were obtained for the components of the CAPSTI: Professional self-concept (PSCNI) (including professional practice, satisfaction and communication); technological influences (TIQ & TIS); and caring attributes (CAQ) (including theoretical, practical, and pedagogical perspectives) (Arthur et al., 1999).

The international sample was derived from an international team of collaborators who were invited to participate in the project via letter. Colleagues in six countries agreed to participate, and later other interested colleagues agreed to participate. Each site was asked to translate the instrument into the local language, to administer the instrument to a randomly selected sample of 250 registered nurses working in a clinical hospital setting, and to send the completed questionnaires to the Hong Kong research team. Eventually 11 countries participated, requiring the instruments to be translated into Chinese and Korean and the results were entered into a comprehensive database for descriptive and inferential analysis.

A total of 1,957 questionnaires from 11 different countries were analyzed. Within the four parts of the scale, Cronbach's alphas were reported as follows: PSCNI .89; TIQ .75; TISQ .94; and CAQ .88. Face and construct validity of the CAPSTI were established from the literature and the original pilot study. Significant correlations were found between and among the different parts of the CAPSTI. Pearson's r correlation coefficients were reported at $P < 0.0001$; between the PSCNI and CAQ ($r = 0.51$); between the PSCNI and TIQ = .13; between the CAQ and the TIQ = .16. Mean scores on the different parts of the instrument differed between and among the various countries. For example, on the caring attribute dimension, the China (Beijing) sample had the lowest mean score; the Philippine sample was significantly different from all but South Africa and Sweden. The Canadian sample was significantly different from the Korean. The items which solicited the highest mean for the total sample were: "Creating a sense of trust"; "A confident relationship between a nurse and a patient is one based on trust, truth, and respect"; "Allowing the patient to express feelings"; "Paying attention to the patient when he/she is talking"; and "Listening to the patient." The exception among the results was that Canadian and South African sample reported the highest scores on "Treating patient's information confidentially." In general, in terms of the caring attributes, all respondents scored greater than 3 on the Likert scale, the arbitrary midpoint of the caring continuum.

The Philippine sample had the highest mean score for caring attributes. Overall, a caring trusting relationship between the nurse and patient was one of the aspects of caring commonly reported among most of the international sample. Additional detailed differences between and among the different countries is reported in the Arthur et al. citation (1999).

This research and instrument is the first of its kind to develop and empirically test and measure caring across different countries. Moreover, it is an ambitious study that has attempted to compare and contrast caring attributes in relation to professional self-concept and technological influences in an international sample. The CAPSTI has been reported to be reliable and valid, helping to create a composite picture of caring through the makeup of nurses in various countries and cultures. The primary author, Arthur (2001) reports that currently there are two studies underway which are using the modified instrument: Korea with a sample of general nurses; Thailand and Hong Kong with a sample of mental health nurses; and with gerontological nurses in Hong Kong and Scotland. In addition, more stringent validation of the instrument is underway through these new studies.

The CAPSTI provides promise for further research and testing, and offers a foundation for future studies across cultures and countries. This instrument is copyrighted by Arthur, who be contacted as noted in the matrix in Table 17.1 which follows.

TABLE 17.1 Matrix of Caring Attributes, Professional Self-Concept and Technological Influences (Arthur, 1998, 1999)

Instrument and Year Developed	Author & Contact Information	Source Citation Publication	Developed to Measure	Instrument Description	Participants	Reported Validity/Reliability	Conceptual-Theoretical Basis of Measurement	Latest Citation in Nursing Literature
Caring attributes professional self-concept—technological influence CAPSTI	David Arthur, Associate Professor, Hong Kong Polytechnic University, Hong Kong, Kowloon, Hong Kong Ph: + 852 2766 6390 Fax: +852 2364 96663 Email: *hsarthur@ inet.polyu. edu.hk*	Arthur, D., Pang, S., Wong, T., Alexander, M. F., et al. (1999). Caring attributes, professional self-concept and technological, influences in a sample of registered nurses in eleven countries. *International Journal of Nursing Studies, 36,* 387–396.	Multidimensional construct of caring internationally	Uses 3 subscales of caring attributes and 3 subscales of PSCNI—13 items theoretical; 41 items practical; 7 items pedagogical	Total sample 1,957 RNs from 11 countries, e.g., Hong Kong, Australia, Canada, China, Korea, New Zealand, Philippines, Scotland, Singapore, South Africa, Sweden	Cronbach's alpha 0.75 overall; PSCNI = 0.89; TIQ = .75; TISQ = .94; CAQ = .88	Items designed to reflect theoretical, practical, and pedagogical perspectives of caring. Items in 3 categories generated by caring theory literature: e.g., Leininger, Benner, Watson; informed by empirical work of Lea & Watson and Wolf	Arthur, D., et al. (1999). Caring attributes, professional self-concept and technological influences in a sample of registered nurses in eleven countries. *International Journal of Nursing Studies, 36,* 387–396. Arthur, D., Pang, S., & Wong, T. (2001). The effects of technology on the caring attributes of an international sample of nurses. *International Journal of Nursing Studies, 38,* 37–43.

CARING ATTRIBUTES PROFESSIONAL SELF-CONCEPT TECHNOLOGICAL INFLUENCE*

DEPARTMENT OF HEALTH SCIENCES NURSING STUDIES SECTION OPINION SURVEY

This questionnaire was developed by nurses from the Department of Health Sciences at the Hong Kong Polytechnic University.

This is an international study involving nurses from different countries including: Australia, Canada, China, Hong Kong, Japan, Macau, the Philippines, Scotland, South Africa, South Korea, and Sweden.

By filling in the questionnaire you will be helping us develop a profile of how nurses in different cultures approach caring and professional issues in nursing.

This questionnaire consists of four parts which explore nurses' perceptions of caring, professional-self and technological influences in their caring practice. In all four parts please express your opinion upon the item statements.

All data will be kept confidential and only group results will be reported. It is not necessary to write your name.

Thank you for taking the time to complete the questionnaire.

Yours sincerely,

David Arthur   Thomas Wong   Samantha Pang

This study is funded by the University Grants Committee of Hong Kong
©*Arthur, Pang, Wong, 1997.*

CARING ATTRIBUTES PROFESSIONAL SELF-CONCEPT TECHNOLOGICAL INFLUENCE
Reprinted by permission of author

PART II

Answer each item by ranking your agreement on the four-point scale: 1 = disagree, 2 = tend to disagree, 3 = tend to agree, 4 = agree. *By circling one symbol ('1' or '4') you are indicating your disagreement or agreement.*

Rank your degree of agreement with the following items. *How well does each item describe you and your work as a nurse:*

Item		1 = disagree	2 = tend to disagree	3 = tend to agree	4 = agree
1.	When I am at work and the situation calls, I am able to think of alternatives.	1	2	3	4
2.	I am a skillful nurse.	1	2	3	4
3.	I am a competent leader.	1	2	3	4
4.	I believe that flexibility is one of my attributes.	1	2	3	4
5.	Competency is one of my characteristics.	1	2	3	4
6.	When I am in charge, people work efficiently.	1	2	3	4
7.	I generally look forward to going to work.	1	2	3	4
8.	When confronted with nursing problems my creativity helps me to solve them.	1	2	3	4
9.	I do not believe I am particularly empathic.	1	2	3	4
10.	Nursing is a rewarding career.	1	2	3	4
11.	Flexibility helps solve nursing problems.	1	2	3	4
12.	I prefer a barrier between me and my patients.	1	2	3	4
13.	I would rather not have the responsibility of leadership.	1	2	3	4
14.	Work as a nurse is generally as I expected before started.	1	2	3	4

Item		1 = disagree	2 = tend to disagree	3 = tend to agree	4 = agree
15.	I am quick to grasp the essentials of nursing problems, to see alternative solutions, and to select the most appropriate solution.	1	2	3	4
16.	I think it is important to share emotions with patients.	1	2	3	4
17.	Most of my colleagues seem willing to work with me as a leader.	1	2	3	4
18.	I regret ever starting nursing.	1	2	3	4
19.	On the whole I am satisfied with my creative approach to my work as a nurse.	1	2	3	4
20.	Competency is the demonstrated ability to successfully apply knowledge and skills in the performance of complex tasks. I am a competent nurse.	1	2	3	4
21.	I feel more comfortable not getting too emotionally close to the people I work with.	1	2	3	4
22.	Decision making is one of my attributes.	1	2	3	4
23.	Nursing is less satisfying than I thought it would be.	1	2	3	4
24.	I usually perform skills as well as my other colleagues.	1	2	3	4
25.	I feel trapped as a nurse.	1	2	3	4
26.	My flexible approach brings out the best in my patients.	1	2	3	4
27.	I think I will continue in nursing for most of my working life.	1	2	3	4
28.	In nursing, it is important to have professional interaction with colleagues.	1	2	3	4
29.	Most people would say nursing is a valuable profession.	1	2	3	4

Item	1 = disagree	2 = tend to disagree	3 = tend to agree	4 = agree
30. I think I am respected as a nurse by other professionals.	1	2	3	4

Item	1 = disagree	2 = tend to disagree	3 = uncertain	4 = tend to agree	5 = agree
31. I don't think there is any more spare time in nursing even though we have an increase in technology.	1	2	3	4	5
32. High technology requires high-tech skills.	1	2	3	4	5
33. The increase in technology in nursing has increased the workload of nurses.	1	2	3	4	5
34. The increase of technical tasks has downgraded the nursing profession.	1	2	3	4	5
35. The influx of technology has raised the profession of nurses.	1	2	3	4	5
36. Due to the application of technology nurses often become frustrated when the inevitable death of a patient occurs.	1	2	3	4	5
37. Technology and the use of machines often interfere with providing adequate nursing care.	1	2	3	4	5
38. Nurses often neglect patients because of the influx of machines.	1	2	3	4	5
39. I'm not sure about the benefits of technology to my practice.	1	2	3	4	5
40. In general technology enhances patient care and well-being.	1	2	3	4	5

Item	1 = disagree	2 = tend to disagree	3 = uncertain	4 = tend to agree	5 = agree
41. Technology has resulted in nurses becoming increasingly professionally uncertain.	1	2	3	4	5
42. Mastery of technology has helped nurses control their work environment.	1	2	3	4	5
43. Technology is an activity which adds meaning to the work of nurses.	1	2	3	4	5
44. Mastery of technology is a useful tool in developing the professional status of nurses.	1	2	3	4	5

PART III

These questions aim to explore your impression of the technological influences in a hospital. Please give your response as quickly as you can.

1. *What is your present working unit?* _____
2. *In your experience as a nurse, how would you rate the technological influence in the following different units of a hospital? Please rate the* **degree of technological influence** *in the following units.*

UNIT	1 = very low	2 = low	3 = moderate	4 = high	5 = very high
Intensive Care Unit (ICU)	1	2	3	4	5
Cardiac Care Unit	1	2	3	4	5
Orthopaedic and Traumatology Unit	1	2	3	4	5
Renal Unit	1	2	3	4	5
Geriatric Unit	1	2	3	4	5
Radiotherapy and Oncology Unit	1	2	3	4	5
Medical Unit	1	2	3	4	5
Surgical Unit	1	2	3	4	5
Neurosurgical Unit	1	2	3	4	5

UNIT	1 = very low	2 = low	3 = moderate	4 = high	5 = very high
Obstetrics Unit	1	2	3	4	5
Labour Room	1	2	3	4	5
Neonatal and Infant Care Unit	1	2	3	4	5
Neonatal ICU	1	2	3	4	5
Paediatric Unit	1	2	3	4	5
Burn Unit	1	2	3	4	5
Infection Control Unit	1	2	3	4	5
Operating Theatre	1	2	3	4	5
Accident and Emergency Department	1	2	3	4	5
General Out-Patient Department	1	2	3	4	5
Specialty Out-Patient Department	1	2	3	4	5
Haematology Unit	1	2	3	4	5
Organ Transplantation Unit	1	2	3	4	5
Psychiatric Unit	1	2	3	4	5
Gynaecology Unit	1	2	3	4	5
Ear, Nose and Throat Unit	1	2	3	4	5
Neurology Unit	1	2	3	4	5
Sport Medicine Unit	1	2	3	4	5
Cardiothoracic Surgery Unit	1	2	3	4	5
Dental Unit	1	2	3	4	5
Ophthalmology Unit	1	2	3	4	5

PART IV

The following items relate to *what caring means to you* as a nurse. Rank your degree of agreement. Try to write what you believe, not what others say, or what others might expect you to say.

Item	1 = disagree	2 = tend to disagree	3 = uncertain	4 = tend to agree	5 = agree
1. Caring is a natural human response and does not require any planning.	1	2	3	4	5
2. Caring is the central feature of nursing.	1	2	3	4	5

Item	1 = disagree	2 = tend to disagree	3 = uncertain	4 = tend to agree	5 = agree
3. Caring nurses are motivated by a feeling or emotion to provide care for patients.	1	2	3	4	5
4. In plain language caring is a 'joint effort' between the nurse and the patient.	1	2	3	4	5
5. Caring is a planned nurse activity designed to meet patient's needs.	1	2	3	4	5
6. Caring is acting, it is not just a feeling.	1	2	3	4	5
7. Caring is a central virtue in nursing and focuses on the nurse as the moral agent.	1	2	3	4	5
8. Caring is aimed at preserving the dignity of the patient.	1	2	3	4	5
9. Caring is unique in nursing.	1	2	3	4	5
10. A nurse cannot care too much.	1	2	3	4	5
11. Caring makes no difference to the patient's health condition.	1	2	3	4	5
12. If a nurse ceases to care, he/she ceases to be a nurse.	1	2	3	4	5
13. Caring is a tool for technology.	1	2	3	4	5

Rank your degree of agreement with the following items. *When I am working with my patient, I am being caring when I am:*

Item		1 = disagree	2 = tend to disagree	3 = uncertain	4 = tend to agree	5 = agree
15.	Being empathic.	1	2	3	4	5
16.	Avoiding the patient.	1	2	3	4	5
17.	Listening to the patient.	1	2	3	4	5
18.	Touching the patient when comfort is needed.	1	2	3	4	5
19.	Allowing the patient to express feelings.	1	2	3	4	5
20.	Talking to the patient.	1	2	3	4	5
21.	Helping to make experiences more pleasant.	1	2	3	4	5
22.	Demonstrating professional skills.	1	2	3	4	5
23.	Putting the needs of the hospital before the patient.	1	2	3	4	5
24.	Communicating with the patient.	1	2	3	4	5
25.	Providing the patient with encouragement.	1	2	3	4	5
26.	Helping the patient clarifying thinking.	1	2	3	4	5
27.	Expecting the patient to do what I tell him/her.	1	2	3	4	5
28.	Treating patient's information confidentially.	1	2	3	4	5
29.	Helping the patient with his/her activities of daily living.	1	2	3	4	5
30.	Giving the patient explanations concerning his/her care.	1	2	3	4	5
31.	When I don't give the patient all the information he/she needs.	1	2	3	4	5
32.	Educating the patient about some aspects of self-care.	1	2	3	4	5
33.	Keeping the relatives informed about the patient as negotiated with the patient.	1	2	3	4	5

Item		1 = disagree	2 = tend to disagree	3 = uncertain	4 = tend to agree	5 = agree
34.	Preventing any anticipated problems/dangers from occurring.	1	2	3	4	5
35.	Knowing what to do in an emergency.	1	2	3	4	5
36.	Creating a sense of trust.	1	2	3	4	5
37.	Speaking up for the patient when it is perceived that something harmful will be done to the patient.	1	2	3	4	5
38.	Speaking on behalf of the patient, in relation to their care.	1	2	3	4	5
39.	Paying attention to the patient when he/she is talking.	1	2	3	4	5
40.	Documenting care given to patient.	1	2	3	4	5
41.	Working collaboratively with colleagues to ensure continuity of care.	1	2	3	4	5
42.	Not involving the patient in the planning of their care.	1	2	3	4	5

Rank your degree of agreement with the following items. *How well does each item describe a caring nurse:*

Item		1 = disagree	2 = tend to disagree	3 = uncertain	4 = tend to agree	5 = agree
43.	To be a caring nurse is to just ask someone how they are, and to look after and provide for them.	1	2	3	4	5
44.	To be a caring nurse is to care for another person and to help him/her.	1	2	3	4	5

Item	1 = disagree	2 = tend to disagree	3 = uncertain	4 = tend to agree	5 = agree
45. To be a caring nurse is to do your best to make someone comfortable in their surroundings.	1	2	3	4	5
46. Caring nurses do not feel concern for the well-being of others.	1	2	3	4	5
47. To be a caring nurse is to help someone who is suffering from a disability and is unable to do things you can do.	1	2	3	4	5
48. A committed nurse is one who is prepared to work extra time with no pay.	1	2	3	4	5
49. The human expression of compassion is a necessary component of caring in an environment which is technologically cold and impersonal.	1	2	3	4	5
50. A competent nurse is someone who has respect for themselves, the profession and patients.	1	2	3	4	5
51. A confident relationship between a nurse and a patient is one based on trust, truth and respect.	1	2	3	4	5
52. A caring nurse is displaying conscience when they are morally aware of their relationship and the status of their actions on others.	1	2	3	4	5
53. A committed nurse is one who balances personal desires and professional obligations to provide care to patients.	1	2	3	4	5

Rank your degree of agreement with how each item describes, *how caring is learned and taught:*

Item	1 = disagree	2 = tend to disagree	3 = uncertain	4 = tend to agree	5 = agree
54. Caring is learned through instruction in counselling techniques.	1	2	3	4	5
55. Caring is learned by modelling in the clinical setting.	1	2	3	4	5
56. Caring cannot be learned or taught.	1	2	3	4	5
57. To care for a patient is an obligation according to patient's needs, regardless of the nurses' experience or ability.	1	2	3	4	5
58. Nurses learn about caring in the nursing school.	1	2	3	4	5
59. Nurses learn about caring by observing other nurses work.	1	2	3	4	5
60. Nurses learn about caring from personal experience.	1	2	3	4	5

END
Thank you for your cooperation.

18

Caring Professional Scale

(Swanson, 2000)

The Caring Professional Scale (CPS) was an investigator-developed (Swanson, 2000) paper-and-pencil questionnaire used in an NIH, NINR research grant (R29 01899) to study how consumers rate health care providers on their practice relationship style. It was developed as a means to evaluate both the nurse and as a way of evaluating the care received from the physician, midwife, and/or nurse at the time a woman was miscarrying a child.

The conceptual-theoretical basis of the scale emerged from Swanson's Caring Theory, an original middle range theory, which was developed over a series of clinical research studies in the area of women's health (Swanson, 1991). The CPS consists of two factor analytically derived subscales: Compassionate Healer and Competent Practitioner. These items were derived from Swanson's original theory categories of:

- Knowing
- Being with
- Doing for
- Enabling
- Maintaining belief

The definition of caring that is grounded in both theory and empirical findings is: Caring is "a nurturing way of relating to a valued other toward whom one feels a personal sense of commitment and responsibility" (Swanson, 1991).

The actual scale consists of 14 items constructed on a 5-point Likert-type scale. Sample items include: Was the provider who just took care of

you . . . comforting? . . . Informative? . . . Technically skilled? . . . Supportive? . . . An attentive listener? . . . Clinically competent? . . . Aware of your
feelings? etc. (Swanson, 2000a). Aside from the empirical development
and evolution of Swanson's Theory, the Caring Professional Scale reliability
and validity were established by correlating the CPS with the empathy
subscale of the Barret-Lennart Relationship Inventory ($r = .61$, $P < 0.001$),
which supports criterion validity (Swanson, 2000a). Cronbach's alpha esti-
mates for internal consistency were used to rate the multiple providers:
advanced practice nurses (.74 to .96), nurses (.97), and physicians (.96).

The sample used for the tool development and testing was a group of
185 women who were participants in a study exploring the effects of caring
(nurse counseling based on Swanson's Caring Theory), measurement
(early versus delayed), passage of time on integration of loss (miscarriage
impact), and emotional well-being (moods and self esteem). The CPS was
developed by the investigator as one strategy to monitor caring as the
intervention/process variable (Swanson, 2000b).

This instrument is unique in that it is designed to be used for assessing
a variety of health professionals on the caring relationship; it is empirically
and theoretically derived by the investigator, and has been used in a
federally funded clinical research investigations whereby caring was the
intervention. The findings from Swanson's intervention study provide evidence that caring was effective as an intervention modality for reducing
emotional disturbance, anger, and depression for women who have miscar-
ried (Swanson, 2000b).

Finally, the original theory from which the CPS emerged has been
found from Swanson's recent meta-analysis (Swanson, 1999) to validate
the generalizability, or transferability, of Swanson's Caring Theory beyond
the perinatal contexts from which it was originally derived. It stands as a
promising caring measurement that has both theoretical and empirical
validity and clinical relevance across settings, populations, and health care
professionals. This instrument is copyrighted and the author request that
she be contacted for permission and advice regarding its use. Table 18.1
provides an overview of key properties of the instrument in a matrix format.

TABLE 18.1 Matrix of Caring Professional Scale (Swanson, 2000)

Instrument & Year Developed	Author & Contact Information	Year Published & Source Citation	Developed to Measure	Instrument Description	Participants	Reported Reliability/Validity	Conceptual-Theoretical Basis of Measurement	Latest Citation in Nursing Literature
Caring Professional Scale (CPS) Swanson (2000a, b)	Dr. Kristine Swanson Professor of Nursing, Chair of Family and Child Nursing, University of Washington, Box 357262, Seattle, WA 98195 Ph: 206-543-8228 FAX 206-543-6656 *kswanson@u.washington.edu*	Swanson, K. (2000a). Predicting depressive symptoms after miscarriage: A path analysis based on the Lazarus Paradigm. *Journal of Women's Health & Gender-Based Medicine, 9*(2), 191–206.	Consumers rating of health care providers on their practice relationship	14-item, 5-point Likert scale; items derived from Swanson's Caring Theory, and empirical research, that reflects Swanson's empirically derived subcategories: -knowing, -being-with, -doing for, -enabling, and -maintaining belief.	185 women who had experienced miscarriage	Construct and content validity through correlation with Barret-Lennart Relationship Inventory subscale of empathy ($r = .61$, $P < 0.001$); Cronbach's alpha (.74 to .96 advanced practice nurses) (.97 for nurses) & (.96 for physicians)	Swanson's Caring Theory a middle range, empirically derived clinical research-based theory and instrument	Swanson, K. (2000b). A program of research on caring. In M. E. Parker (Ed.), *Nursing Theories and Nursing Practice.* Philadelphia: F. A. Davis NIH, NINR, R29 01899, UW Centre for Women's Health Research, NIH, NINR, P30 NR04001

CARING PROFESSIONAL SCALE*

DIRECTIONS: Circle the number under the words that best describe the way experienced your health care provider.

	Yes, Definitely	Mostly	About Half and Half	Occasionally	No, Not at All	Not Applicable
Was the Health Care Provider that just took care of you:						
1. Emotionally distant?	1	2	3	4	5	N/A
2. Comforting?	1	2	3	4	5	N/A
3. Positive?	1	2	3	4	5	N/A
4. Abrupt?	1	2	3	4	5	N/A
5. Insulting?	1	2	3	4	5	N/A
6. Informative?	1	2	3	4	5	N/A
7. Clinically competent?	1	2	3	4	5	N/A
8. Understanding?	1	2	3	4	5	N/A
9. Personal?	1	2	3	4	5	N/A
10. Caring?	1	2	3	4	5	N/A
11. Supportive?	1	2	3	4	5	N/A
12. An attentive listener?	1	2	3	4	5	N/A
13. Centered on you?	1	2	3	4	5	N/A
14. Technically skilled?	1	2	3	4	5	N/A
15. Aware of your feelings?	1	2	3	4	5	N/A
16. Visibly touched by your experience?	1	2	3	4	5	N/A
17. Able to offer you hope?	1	2	3	4	5	N/A
18. Respectful of you?	1	2	3	4	5	N/A

©Swanson, 2001.

---

*©Kristen M. Swanson. Reprinted by permission of the author.

19

Methodist Health Care System
Nurse Caring Instrument

(Shepherd, Sherwood et al., 2000)

This tool, referred to as the Methodist Health Care System Nurse Caring Instrument (MHCSNCI), was developed by the Nursing Quality Indicator Caring Subcommittee at Methodist Health Care System in Houston, Texas. The Subcommittee members include: Mary Shepherd, RN, MS, CNAA, Gwen Sherwood, PhD, RN, Mari Rude, RN, MS, CS, AOCN, and Lillian Eriksen, DSN, RN. This tool emerged from the nursing leadership team and a system-wide Nursing Quality Indicator Committee which was concerned with quality indicators for which nursing would hold itself accountable. The Committee identified *nurses' caring* as a key indicator. The tool development was incorporated into an academic and clinical partnership between The Methodist Hospital and The University of Texas School of Nursing in Houston. Thus, an outcome-based research study of nurses' caring became part of the initiative that generated the Nurse Caring Instrument.

The MHCSNCI was designed to measure patient satisfaction with caring. The conceptual-theoretical basis of the instrument reflects a range of contemporary caring literature and concepts from different caring theories. Items and dimensions were identified from a qualitative approach to content analysis from 42 literature citations. The result generated 12 dominant and 14 supportive dimensions of caring that became the core of the project. Content validity was achieved through focus groups of 200 Methodist nurses who identified 51 dimensions of caring. These were cross-referenced with the literature. Two focus groups of 21 patients further validated the final 12 dominant dimensions of caring that had been identified. The 12 dominant dimensions included such areas as: care coordination, competence, teaching/learning, emotional support, respect for individuality, physical comfort, availability, helping/trusting relationship, patient/family involvement, physical environment, spiritual environment, outcomes. The items are reflective of concepts from the caring literature and caring theory of Watson and others, as well as items that are familiar areas of assessment reflected on other instruments.

The purpose for the specific process of instrument development was to develop a valid and reliable instrument, to test its psychometric properties for measuring patient satisfaction with nurses' caring, and to establish a baseline for measuring future changes. Instrument testing included a sample of 369 medical-surgical patients who received, and responded to, a 33-item instrument through the mail. From that sample the scale was refined to 20 items. An Intra-Class Correlation yielded an ICC of .98 with no interaction effect. Construct validity was established through a principal axis factoring with a varimax rotation. One factor emerged which accounted for 75% of the variance. Additional validity was apparent in mean scores for patient care units. For example, units expected to score higher on the scale did, indeed, report the highest mean scores.

Additional repeat measurements and refinements of the tool are underway. A repeat measure is planned to re-evaluate caring-based outcomes. This repeat measure is to follow a year-long, system-wide educational intervention for creating a caring community, including practice guidelines and performance indicators for standards of care for the nursing staff at Methodist Health Care System.

The MHCSNCI is a first-generation caring assessment tool, but has been tested with over 300 patients. It consists of 20 items on a Likert-type scale, informed by content analysis of caring literature. Because of the infancy of this instrument, there are no publication sources at this time. However, the development and testing of the instrument and findings to date have been presented at two inter/national conferences (Shepherd & Sherwood, 1999; Shepherd et al., 2001). Further analysis, testing and validation for the instrument are underway and continuing. The Methodist Hospital holds the copyright for the instrument and offers support for its ongoing refinement and use. The authors encourage anyone interested to contact them directly. Table 19.1 provides a matrix that includes key information regarding the evolution and development of the Methodist Health Care System Nurse Caring Instrument to date.

TABLE 19.1 Matrix of Methodist Health Care System Nurse Caring Instrument (Sherwood & Shepherd, 1999, 2000)

Instrument and Year Developed	Author and Contact Address	Publication Source Citation	Developed to Measure	Instrument Description	Participants	Reported Reliability/ Validity	Conceptual-Theoretical Basis of Measurement	Latest Citation in Nursing Literature
Methodist Health Care System Nurse Caring Instrument (MHCSNCI)	Mary Shepherd, RN, MSN, CNAA Director, Methodist Health Care System, 6565 Fannin Street, Houston, Texas 77030-2707 Ph: 713-790 2531 *MLShepherd@tmh.tmc.edu* Dr. Gwen Sherwood Professor of Nursing, University of Texas-Houston, Health Sciences Center, School of Nursing, Houston, Texas FAX: 713 500 2026 *gsherwoo@son1.nur.uth.tmc.edu*	Unpublished to date, 2001	Valid and reliable instrument of nurses' caring; to operationalize caring as a core concept in patient satisfaction and outcome-based research on nurses' caring	20-item Likert-type scale; measures dominant components of caring	n = 200 nurses; 21 patients; revised version to sample of n = 369 medical-surgical patients	Intra-Class Correlation 0.98; Construct validity with principal axis factoring with varimax rotation Content validity with staff nurses	Empirically derived from multiple views of caring in the nursing literature; qualitative content analysis	None to date; Two formal research presentations: Shepherd & Sherwood, 1999 Sigma Theta Tau International 35th Biennial convention; Shepherd et al. (2000) International Association for Human Caring Research Conference

THE METHODIST HEALTH CARE SYSTEM NURSE CARING INSTRUMENT*

Directions: Please assist us in evaluating our nursing services by reading the following descriptions. For each description CIRCLE the ONE NUMBER that BEST shows your opinion about the nursing care you received during your most recent hospital admission.

The nursing staff:	Seldom or Rarely		Often or Frequent			Always or Almost Always		Does Not Apply
1. Communicated a helping and trusting attitude (Helping/Trusting)	1	2	3	4	5	6	7	
2. Considered my needs when scheduling procedures or medications (Individual Respect)	1	2	3	4	5	6	7	
3. Offered me a choice regarding my treatment plan (Individual Respect)	1	2	3	4	5	6	7	
4. Helped me understand the changes in my life from my illness (Helping/Trusting)	1	2	3	4	5	6	7	
5. Involved me in my care (Patient Involvement)	1	2	3	4	5	6	7	
6. Involved my family and significant others in my care (Family Involvement)	1	2	3	4	5	6	7	
7. Made me feel that if I needed nursing care again, I would come back to this hospital (Outcome)	1	2	3	4	5	6	7	

*©The Methodist Hospital, Houston, Texas. Instrument developed by the Nursing Quality Indicator Subcommittee under the direction of Mary Shepherd, RN, MSN, CNAA. Reprinted with permission.

The nursing staff:	Seldom or Rarely		Often or Frequent			Always or Almost Always		Does Not Apply
8. Made me feel secure when giving me care (Emotional Support)	1	2	3	4	5	6	7	
9. Made spiritual care and resources available to me (Spiritual)	1	2	3	4	5	6	7	
10. Made sure other staff knew how to care for me (Care Coordination)	1	2	3	4	5	6	7	
11. Provided basic comfort measures (Physical Environment)	1	2	3	4	5	6	7	
12. Demonstrated professional knowledge and skills (Competence)	1	2	3	4	5	6	7	
13. Provided good physical care (Physical Comfort)	1	2	3	4	5	6	7	
14. Recognized that I may have special needs (Care Coordination)	1	2	3	4	5	6	7	
15. Returned to check on me, not just when I called (Availability)	1	2	3	4	5	6	7	
16. Showed concern for me (Emotional Support)	1	2	3	4	5	6	7	
17. Taught me to care for myself whenever appropriate (Teaching/Learning)	1	2	3	4	5	6	7	
18. Took care of my requests in a reasonable time (Availability)	1	2	3	4	5	6	7	

The nursing staff:	Seldom or Rarely		Often or Frequent			Always or Almost Always		Does Not Apply
19. Were honest with me (Helping/Trusting)	1	2	3	4	5	6	7	
20. Were pleasant and friendly to me (Helping/Trusting)	1	2	3	4	5	6	7	

Comments :

_____

_____

_____

PART III

Challenges and Future Directions

20

The Evolution of Measuring Caring: Moving Toward Construct Validity

Carolie Coates

THE CHALLENGE OF ASSESSING CARING: DIFFICULT, BUT NOT IMPOSSIBLE

Nurses have described a major part of what they do, in both historical and contemporary works, as "caring" (Kyle, 1995; Lea & Watson, 1996; McCance, McKenna, & Boore, 1997; Morse, Solberg, Neander, Bottorff, & Johnson, 1990). While this aspect of the nursing role has been almost universally accepted, some nurses and their critics have argued that caring is so elusive it cannot be captured and documented. This stance is no longer very defensible or functional. In the current cost-conscious, rapidly changing health care world, to refuse or to ignore the need to document and to measure the effects of a foundational aspect of one's professional role (e.g., caring), may signal to other professions the lack of importance, value, or even existence of the concept of nurse caring.

Psychologists and other social scientists have taken up the challenge of quantitative assessment of similarly complex and daunting personal constructs like empathy, self-esteem, empowerment, anxiety, self-efficacy, and locus of control with good success. Similarly, psychologists, educational psychologists, and other measurement specialists have responded to the need to devise measures relevant to social relationships including social support, reciprocity, powerlessness, leadership style, learning style, and parenting style. Currently a number of measures with strong validity and reliability markers are available to assess all of these constructs.

The assessment of the construct of caring is similar in that it, too, is difficult to operationally define, is multifaceted, and encompasses complexities of human interaction. Caring is particularly difficult to assess because it entails a *dynamic process* that involves, at minimum, not only the nurse or health care provider, but also an "other," the patient. The most frequently used approach has examined nurse caring as a set of behaviors, for example Larson, Wolf, Cronin, and Harrison (date). Some have turned their attention to assessing the nature of the caring relationship of nurse-patient, caring as the quality of a relationship or confidence that one can achieve a caring relationship, e.g., Coates (1997). Others, like Hughes (1993), have focused on the features of an organizational or educational climate that exemplify caring. Some caring scale developers such as Nkongo (1990) have focused on the ability of the nurse to deliver caring.

The purpose of this chapter is to examine the progress that nurses and members of related disciplines have made in defining and measuring caring in health care. For as Fitzpatrick (1995) reminds us in her editorial, "Where has all the caring gone?", nursing research should be a force to restore balance in the health care system so that it is not totally cost-driven. Despite the difficulties in definition and measurement, nursing needs to continue the work that was begun to explore and assess the nature of caring and its effects on practice and health outcomes. If caring is valued, we must define and assess it with credibility, and not always let quality of patient care and caring take a secondary or tertiary position to the premium placed by the health care marketplace on assessing the costs of health care.

Kyle (1995) summarized the position of two qualitatively oriented researchers, Leininger and Ray, who in the 1980s criticized the early quantitative measurement studies as " . . . impeding the study of care . . . " (p. 510). Thus, there is a position held by some qualitative researchers that the quantitative researchers should hold off until qualitative researchers have sufficiently investigated the meaning and mapping of the concept of caring. While qualitative research on caring has made tremendous strides in exploring the meaning and culture of caring, most do not claim that they have accomplished an exhaustive exploration or mapping of the concept of caring. Knowledge can be advanced by qualitatively and quantitatively focused research, as well as by studies using blended designs. This is too new a research enterprise to put limits on the type of research that is appropriate.

However, the complex scene of quantitative caring measures resembles a patchwork quilt, with more and more measures being developed, but almost none of them being used concurrently or with similar populations. This complexity and proliferation of studies that do not overlap in the definition of caring, the use of measurement tools, or samples, provides a confusing scene for investigators hoping to include the concept of caring in the scope of their research. Even Lea and Watson, who are committed to quantitative study of caring, have commented on the confusion resulting from the addition of more and more quantitative studies to assess caring. They stress the need to reduce caring to its underlying dimensions in order to better understand the structure of the concept (Lea & Watson, 1996, p. 75).

NEW CONCEPTION OF VALIDITY

Nursing research has embraced traditional standards of reliability and validity to assess the rigor of quantitative instruments (Burns & Grove, 2001; Polit & Hungler, 1999). Jacobson (1997) developed a very thorough chapter which outlines the psychometric criteria used to evaluate the quality of instruments for use in clinical research. Seminal works on issues in measurement are cited, for example, in Waltz, Strickland, and Lenz (1991). The traditional psychometric criteria of reliability (as stability, as equivalence, or as internal consistency) and validity (face, content, criterion-related, or construct validity) have been defined. Jacobson (1997) has discussed other desirable characteristics of the instruments including sensitivity (instrument capable of making fine discriminations), appropriateness, objectivity, and feasibility. Nunnally and Bernstein (1994) have suggested that more relaxed psychometric standards be applied as criteria to judge early and later-stage instrument development.

Goodwin (1997) has presented an informative historical review of measurement validity, highlighted by the definitions espoused by key educational and psychological measurement specialists. She summarized the evolution of the meaning of validity over the past 50 years, which brings some fresh insights to the issue of measurement validity for nursing instruments. In the 1940s the emphasis was on determining the validity of a particular test, no matter what its use. In the 1950s through the 1970s, interpretation became closely tied to the use or aim of a specific test. The three-part definition of validity in terms of content, criterion-related, and construct validity provided the standards. Issues of convergent validity (measures a test should theoretically relate to) and discriminant validity (measures a test theoretically should not relate to) took the forefront as methodologies to determine a test's validity. In the 1980s validity was broadened to include the decisions emanating from the test scores. Validation was a process of accumulating evidence to make decisions of social consequence.

In the 1980s there was a shift away from the three-part definition of validity. "More and more, construct validity is seen as the unifying and key meaning of validity" (Goodwin, 1997, p. 103). "Validity is a unitary concept, although various kinds of evidence—typically referred to as content, criterion-related, and construct—need to be sought for a measure" (Goodwin, 1997, p. 103). Construct validity is seen as the overarching concept. Validity is not an all-or-none characteristic, but " . . . a matter of degree . . . " (Goodwin, 1997, p. 104). The instrument is examined with regard to its use in making inferences about group differences, the structure of the measure, and the consequences of using the measure.

Goodwin (1997) pointed out that the conceptualization of instrument reliability is also changing. Traditionally, reliability (consistency) was seen as a separate precursor to validation. In more recent approaches, reliability is conceptualized as part of the study of an instrument's degree of construct validity. In summary, "Today, there is general agreement that validity refers to the degree of accuracy and appropriateness of inferences made from scores, is a unitary concept, is a matter of degree rather than an absolute, all-or-nothing determination, and requires multiple types of evidence before a judgment can be made regarding the validity of a measure for a particular use or interpretation" (Goodwin, 1997, p. 106).

Goodwin (1997) challenges researchers interested in improving measurement in nursing: "Obtaining meaningful validity evidence, to support the inferences to be drawn from scores, is one of the greatest challenges for instrument developers" (p. 107). In an accompanying review, Stewart & Archbold (1997) are supportive of Goodwin's message as it relates to nursing education. They support the dynamic process of pursuing construct validation through multiple studies that challenge the test developer to move back and forth between conceptualization and measurement. They urge researchers to be open to unexpected findings and to emergent interpretations based on many different studies. "Don't be overconfident about your measures until you have used them in multiple studies" (Stewart & Archbold, 1997, p. 101).

REVIEWS OF QUANTITATIVE APPROACHES
TO CARING ASSESSMENT

As context for assessing the measurement work on caring, Jacobson (1997) cited classic reviews of nursing research articles from the early 1980s which concluded that the general state of measurement in nursing was lacking at that time. Critiques called for more emphasis on established measurement principles and practices. She also reiterated what other reviewers have stressed, that many nursing tools reported in published articles cite very small samples, which are less representative and hence have associated findings that are less statistically stable than larger samples. This background information on the state of the art of measurement in nursing in the 1980s is very relevant because the first generation of scales to assess caring were published in the mid to late 1980s, and thus are prone to some of same criticisms of small sample sizes and uneven application of the principles of rigorous instrument development.

A number of excellent reviews of quantitative caring instruments were published in the late 1990s. Kyle (1995) reviewed the three best known instruments at that time: CARE-Q (Larson), CBI (Wolf), and CBA (Cronin and Harrison), as well as a number of major qualitative studies. Kyle warned about the dangers in the quantitative work of studying caring out of context, and the limitations of studying caring when reduced to a preselected list of behaviors. Kyle speculated on possible reasons why nurses tend to identify expressive behaviors as indicators of care more frequently than patients, while patients tend to identify instrumental nursing behaviors more frequently than nurses. Lea and Watson (1996) summarized psychometric properties of two of the same instruments reviewed by Kyle (1995), the CARE-Q and the CBI. Lea and Watson concluded by supporting Valentine's (1991) argument for the need for a large multivariate study which would conceptualize and measure caring as a therapeutic intervention and also explore the relationship of caring to basic demographic variables.

Andrews, Daniels, and Hall (1996) reviewed the psychometric properties of five caring tools: Larson's CARE-Q and CARE/SAT, Nyberg's CAS, Duffy's CAT, and Wolf's CBI. The study was interesting in that it was also a descriptive study that administered these five instruments to the same sample; unfortunately the sample only totaled 26. The small sample size and the diverse structures and scoring methods made the study of relationships among the different instruments "impossible" (Andrews et al., 1996, p. 34). They concluded that the CBI was the most user-friendly caring tool.

Beck (1999) produced a well-organized review of 11 caring instruments identified from the CINAHL database for works published from 1982–1997: CARE-Q (Larson), CBA (Cronin and Harrison), CBI (Wolf), CDI (Watson and Lea), HCI (Latham), CARE/SAT (Larson and Ferketich), CAI (Nkongho), CAS (Nyberg), CPCS (McDaniel), CBC (McDaniel), and CBNS (Hinds). Instruments were reviewed with regard to a number of important characteristics including definition of caring, type of measure, number of items, concept being measured, type of respondents, average time to administer, sample size and types of samples studied, reliability, readability, and validity. Beck concluded that most instruments achieved acceptable reliability levels, but further testing of psychometric properties was needed with larger sample sizes and diverse populations. Methods to address degree of construct validity have been very limited, with factor analysis being the primary method.

Swanson (1999) reviewed both qualitative and quantitative approaches to assessing caring using her framework of five levels: capacity for caring, concerns/commitments, conditions, caring actions, and caring consequences. Level IV: Caring Actions, includes a review of quantitative measures that focus on caring behaviors: CARE-Q, CBA, CBI, SNBC, and Swanson's CPS. Swanson does a masterful job of analyzing the content domains addressed by these scales. She concluded: "The clearest limitation to the study of Level IV caring actions is the lack of controlled clinical trials wherein protocols for caring-based therapeutic interventions are defined, applied, carefully monitored, and tested for effectiveness in promoting health outcomes" (Swanson, 1999, p. 52).

While all of these reviews have added to our understanding of the major caring measurement tools, most of them have not systematically reviewed each instrument with regard to meeting established psychometric standards for instrument development, with the exception of Beck (1999). They have not compared them with regard to their journeys toward construct validity.

EVALUATIVE CRITERIA FOR DEGREE OF CONSTRUCT VALIDITY

TWENTY-ONE QUANTITATIVE CARING MEASURES

Watson's compilation in this volume includes: Larson's Caring Assessment Instrument (CARE-Q) and Caring Satisfaction Questionnaire (CARE/SAT), Wolf's Caring Behavior Inventory (CBI), Cronin and Harrison's Caring Behaviors Assessment (CBA), Hind's Caring Behaviors of Nurses Scale (CBNS), Horner's Professional Caring Behaviors (PCB), Nyberg's Caring Assessment or Caring Attributes Scale (CAS), Nkongho's Caring Ability Inventory (CAI), McDaniel's Caring Behaviors Checklist (CBC) and Client Perception of Caring Scale (CPC), Duffy's Caring Assessment Tool (CAT) and (CAT-admin) version to assess nurses' perceptions of their managers for administrative nursing research, and (CAT-edu) version for educational use, Hughes' Peer Group Caring Interaction Scale (PGCIS) and Organizational Climate for Caring Questionnaire (OCCQ), Coates' Caring Efficacy Scale (CES), Latham's Holistic Caring Inventory (HCI), Watson and Lea's Caring Dimensions Inventory (CDI), Arthur et al.'s Caring Attributes, Professional Self-Concept Technological Influences Scale

(CAPSTI), Swanson's Caring Professional Scale (CPS), and Shepherd and Sherwood, et al.'s Methodist Health Care System Nursing Caring Instrument (MHCSNCI). This inclusive list of 21 caring measures includes the first generation caring tools and their process of refinement (which have been reviewed by others), as well as scales that are not as well known and/or have been developed more recently. The similarity in acronyms alone makes the task of distinguishing one tool from another confusing.

A PROCESS FOR ASSESSING CONSTRUCT VALIDITY

As Watson stated earlier in this volume, most of the scales evolved through the work of one researcher or a small group of investigators working with an individualistic operational definition of caring (sometimes rooted in nursing theory and sometimes not). Most of the investigators were not funded with external research grants and often forced by circumstances to utilize small convenience samples in their initial scale development work. Profiling degree of construct validity for each measure represents a complex organizational challenge at best. A search was made for a rating scheme, which would facilitate application of the same evaluative criteria for construct validity to the psychometric information available for each tool. Application of the evaluative criteria is not meant to imply that one scale is better than another, only to provide some rough markers of the evolutionary and often eclectic journey of each scale. Some of the newer scales have simply not had the time to move very far along the path toward construct validity. Such a systematic application of criteria also permits a view across the current field of caring tool contenders in a holistic way to try to assess the state of the art of caring assessment.

A scheme for applying a set of psychometric criteria to evaluate the degree of construct validity of research instruments was selected and adapted from a method to evaluate attitude measures (Robinson, Shaver, & Wrightsman, 1991). For each evaluative criteria, they suggest rating anchors from 4 to 0, with the larger number indicating more rigor: 4 = exemplary, 3 = extensive, 2 = moderate, 1 = minimal, 0 = none or very limited. In very few instances NA was used to represent "not applicable" because the nature of the scale prohibited the criterion information from being generated. In a few cases the source document was not available to the author and so the rating could not be completed; in these cases the rating is left blank. All of the criteria from Robinson et al. (1991) were included except inter-item correlations and freedom from response set, because data relevant to these concepts tended not to be reported in nursing caring tool articles. The criterion of predictive validity was added. The original scale had strength of theoretical linkage and/or content validity in the same criterion scale. Modification was made so that degree of theoretical linkages to caring theories and strength of content validity testing were split into two separate criteria. In some cases, the anchor descriptions for "exemplary," "extensive," etc., were modified. Please note that the rating process is limited in that only the chapter author made the rating, based on available published source documents. Note that the anchor definitions sometimes call for "fine" distinctions on the 4–0 point scale and not just presence or absence of a criterion. The table is intended as a general guide to give the reader a sense of the state of instrument development as a whole, and is not a report card for any particular instrument. Also, instrument authors may likely have additional relevant unpublished psychometric information that was not included in this rating. (See Table 20.1.)

TABLE 20.1   Application of Rating Criteria to Caring Instruments

CARING SCALE	Caring Theory	Content Validity	Pilot Testing	Samples	Norms	Alpha (Internal Consistency)
1. CARE-Q Larson, 1984	1	4	2	4	4 (ranks)	4 (lower for 1 subscale)
2. CARE/SAT Larson & Fer- ketich, 1993	1	3	2	0	3	4
3. CBI Wolf, 1986, 1994	3	4	2	3	3	4
4. CBA Cronin & Har- rison, 1988	4	2	1	3	3	4 (lower for 2 subscales)
5. CBNS Hinds, 1988	2	2	1	1	3	4
6. PCB Horner, 1989, 1991	1	2	1	1	0	4
7. CAS Nyberg, 1990	4	1	0	0	0	4
8. CAI Nkongho, 1990	4	3	2	2	3	3
9. CBC McDaniel, 1990	1	2	0	0	0	0

TABLE 20.1   *(continued)*

CARING SCALE	Caring Theory	Content Validity	Pilot Testing	Samples	Norms	Alpha (Internal Consistency)
10. CPC McDaniel, 1990	1	2	0	0	0	4
11. CAT Duffy, 1992	3	2	3	1	2	4
12. CAT-A Duffy, rev. 1993	3	2	2	0	2	4
13. CATedu Duffy, 2001	3		2	0	2	4
14. PGCIS Hughes, 1993	1	1	2	2	0	4
15. OCCQ Hughes, 1993	4	2	2	2	0	4
16. CES Coates, 1995, 1997	3	2	1	2	3	4
17. HCI Latham, 1988, 1996	3	2	1	1	3	4
18. CDI Watson & Lea, 1997	1	2	1	2	3	4
19. CAPSTI Arthur et al., 1998, 1999	1	2	3	4	4	4
20. CPS Swanson, 2000	4	2		3	3	4
21. MHCSNCI Sherwood & Shepherd, 2000	1	3	1	2	1	4

(continued)

TABLE 20.1   *(continued)*

CARING SCALE	Factor Analysis	Test-Retest Reliability	Known Groups Validity	Convergent/Divergent Validity	Discriminant Validity	Predictive Validity
1. CARE-Q Larson, 1984	NA-ranked data	4	4	0	0	0
2. CARE/SAT Larson & Ferketich, 1993	2	0	0	1	0	0
3. CBI Wolf, 1986, 1994	4	4	2	0	0	0
4. CBA Cronin & Harrison, 1988	2	4	0	0	0	0
5. CBNS Hinds, 1988	0	0	0	1	0	0
6. PCB Horner, 1989, 1991	0	4	0	0	0	0
7. CAS Nyberg, 1990	0	0	0	0	0	0
8. CAI Nkongho, 1990	2	3	3	1	0	0
9. CBC McDaniel, 1990	0	(appropriate inter-rater reliability)	0	0	0	0
10. CPC McDaniel, 1990	0	0	0	0	0	0
11. CAT Duffy, 1992	0	0	0	1	0	0
12. CAT-A Duffy, rev. 1993	0	0	0	1	0	0
13. CATedu Duffy, 2001	0	0	0	3	0	0
14. PGCIS Hughes, 1993	2	0	0	3	0	0

TABLE 20.1   *(continued)*

CARING SCALE	Factor Analysis	Test-Retest Reliability	Known Groups Validity	Convergent/ Divergent Validity	Discriminant Validity	Predictive Validity
15. OCCQ Hughes, 1993	2	0	0	4	0	0
16. CES Coates, 1995, 1997	2	0	0	4	0	0
17. HCI Latham, 1988, 1996	0	0	0	2	0	0
18. CDI Watson & Lea, 1997	0	0	0	2	0	0
19. CAPSTI Arthur et al., 1998, 1999	0	0	0	4	0	0
20. CPS Swanson, 2000	0	0	0	1	0	0
21. MHCSNCI Sherwood & Shepherd, 2002	2	0	1	0	0	0

Table legend: 4 = Exemplary, 3 = Extensive, 2 = Moderate, 1 = Minimal, and 0 = None or very limited. NA = rating not applicable to instrument. Missing ratings occurred because source documents were not available to rate.

Theoretical Linkage to Caring Theory

This criterion refers to the degree the instrument is anchored in a theoretical framework with its major focus on caring. A rating of 4 means the instrument has strong theoretical linkages to a caring theory, that items and/or subscales were developed from theoretical principles. A 3 means a caring theory was cited as foundational to the instrument development, but it is not spelled out how the theory influenced development of specific items or subscales. A rating of 2 means there are clear linkages to a related theory, but not to one of the theories of caring. A rating of 1 means the general caring literature was cited as a context for instrument development. A rating of 0 means that no theories or literature were cited in relation to development of the instrument.

Content Validity

This criterion is defined as the degree to which the instrument underwent content validity verification during the instrument development phase. Note that this criterion uses a fairly narrow definition of content validity as verification through external expert panels or informed sources. (Factor analysis is rated as a separate criterion, and so is excluded from this consideration of content validity.) A rating of 4 indicates exemplary content validity, i.e., several large empirical studies were conducted with defined samples used to validate test items. A rating of 3 indicates extensive content validity verification, i.e., items were rated by several small groups of content experts or informed sources. A rating of 2 indicates that items were rated by a few content experts or derived from the research literature. A rating of 1 indicates minimal or low level of content validity exemplified only by face validity of the items. A rating of 0 indicates no evidence of any type of content validity verification through ratings by external sources.

Pilot Testing

This criterion refers to use of pilot testing to develop the instrument, and the extensiveness of the original item pool. A rating of 4 means that more than 250 items were in the initial pool and several pilot studies were conducted. A rating of 3 means that 101–250 items were in the initial pool and a pilot study was conducted. A rating of 2 means that 50–100 items were in the initial pool and a pilot study was conducted. A rating of 1 means that some items were eliminated from the original set and a small pilot study conducted. A rating of 0 means that all initial items were included in the scale and no pilot study was conducted.

Samples

This criterion refers to the nature and relative size of the instrument development study samples. A rating of 4 means that large, national or international samples have been utilized. A rating of 3 means that the scale has been tested with several large, diverse samples. A rating of 2 means that several studies have been conducted using moderate size samples. A rating of 1 means that the scale has been used with several convenience group samples. A rating of 0 means that only one convenience group sample has been utilized.

Norms

This criterion refers to the descriptive statistics provided for the scale with regard to various samples or subgroups. A rating of 4 indicates that means and standard deviations are reported for many different samples. A rating of 3 can be interpreted that means and standard deviations are available for several samples. A rating of 2 refers to a situation where means were reported for some groups. A rating of 1 refers to a situation where means were available for only one group. A rating of 0 on this criterion means that no means or standard deviations were reported for any of the groups.

Alpha

Alpha or Cronbach's alpha is a measure of internal consistency of the instrument. A rating of 4 means an overall scale alpha of .80 or better, a rating of 3 refers to an alpha ranging between .70 and .79, a rating of 2 refers to an alpha ranging between .60 and .69 (acceptable for newly developed scales), a rating of 1 means that the reported alpha was below .60, and a rating of 0 means that no alpha calculations were reported for the scale. (If some subscale alphas are low (in the .60s), this was noted in the table. If alphas were reported from more than one study, the most representative rating category was selected.)

Factor Analysis

A rating of 4 means that a factor analysis has been conducted in several studies confirming a similar factor structure. A rating of 3 means that a factor analysis has been conducted on at least two samples. A rating of 2 means that a factor analysis has been performed on at least one sample, with factors accounting for a significant amount of the variance. A rating of 1 indicates that a factor analysis was mentioned with no statistical details. A rating of 0 means that no factor analysis of the scale has been reported.

Test-Retest Reliability

This statistical analysis tests the stability of a test over time, typically 2–4 weeks (Jacobson, 1997, p. 7). A rating of 4 means that scale scores correlate .80 or better. A rating of 3 means that scale scores correlate between .70 and .79. A rating of 2 means that scale scores correlate .60–.69. A rating of 1 means that scale scores correlate less than .60. A rating of 0 means that no test-retest reliability studies are reported. (If test-retest information was available from more than one study, the most representative rating was selected. In the case of instruments that involve ratings by more than one rater or observer, inter-rater reliability (reliability as equivalence) is noted in the table.)

Known Groups Validity

This is a more sophisticated test of whether the scale is demonstrating some degree of "known" groups or "contrasted" group's validity, that is, the ability of the scale to demonstrate statistical significance between two groups known to be high and low on the assessed concept. A rating of 4 means the scale discriminates between known groups in predictable and highly significant ways and that many pairs of known groups have been compared. A rating of 3 indicates that the scale discriminates between several known groups in predictable and highly significant ways. A rating of 2 means that the scale can discriminate between at least two pairs of known groups in predictable ways. A rating of 1 indicates that the scale has discriminated between at least two known groups in predictable ways. A rating of 0 means that no known groups data could be found for the scale.

Convergent/Divergent Validity

This criterion involves obtaining results from use of a scale consistent with theoretical predictions, for example, a related measure that is significantly positively related with the caring scale (demonstrating convergent validity) or an unrelated measure that is significantly negatively correlated with the caring scale (divergent validity) as predicted from theory. This approach assumes the other measures have adequate evidence of reliability and validity. Inferences about relationships of the target scale with other variables are provided. A rating of 4 means that highly significant correlations in predictable directions have been reported with more than 4 measures. A rating of 3 means that significant correlations were found with more than 3 measures. A rating of 2 means correlations reported with two measures. A rating of 1 means correlation with one measure. A rating of 0 means no significant correlations were reported. (Related terms: If the correlation of the caring measure in question involves correlation with another caring measure or criterion measure, the validity assessment is often called criterion-related validity. If the caring measure in question is correlated with another criterion measure given in the same administration, the type of validity is often termed concurrent validity.)

Discriminant Validity

While some researchers tend to treat divergent and discriminant validity as the same, discriminant validity is defined in a particular way for use as a criterion in this analysis of caring instruments. This is a more sophisticated standard of construct validity determined through use of the multitrait-multimethod matrix devised by Campbell and Fiske (1959). "The method requires more than one index of each of several constructs (say x, y, and z) one wants to measure with the instrument. It is best to include as many measures or indices of each construct as possible, as well as to measure for control purposes such variables as intelligence or response set that could also explain apparent relationships. In the resulting correlation matrix, the various items measuring each single construct (say x) should first correlate highly among themselves; second, the correlations among these items should be higher than their correlations with the items intended to measure constructs y or z, or any of the control variables. The latter is evidence of the scale's ability to discriminate from these other measures" (Robinson et al., 1991, p. 14). This very high standard of construct validity remains fairly rare in the nursing literature and in the measurement literature in general. A rating of 4 was given if four discriminant validity studies were conducted, a 3 if three were conducted, a 2 if two were conducted, a 1 if one was conducted, and 0 if none were reported.

Predictive Validity

This criterion refers to predictive studies using the caring scale as a predictor of performance on another measure at some future date. A large sample would be needed and regression would be the likely statistical analysis. A rating of 4 indicates that four or more predictive studies have been conducted, a rating of 3 indicates that three have been conducted, a rating of 2 indicates that two have been conducted, a rating of 1 indicates than one has been conducted, and a rating of 0 indicates that the scale has not been used as a predictor variable in any studies reviewed.

APPRAISAL OF CONSTRUCT VALIDITY OF CARING INSTRUMENTS

Review of the information presented in Table 20.1 leads one to the following conclusions about the state of the art with regard to quantitative measurement in caring:

1. The majority of instruments are theoretically linked but a considerable number were more empirically derived.
2. Most scales have established a reasonable level of content validity.
3. Pilot development of the scales is hampered by relatively small items pools and small convenience group samples.

4. Too often studies neglect to report means and standard deviations for different groups.

5. Reasonably high levels of internal consistency (alpha) have been established for most scales; however, some researchers neglect to calculate alpha in additional studies which utilize the instrument, and simply rely on the original information about the instrument's alpha from the scale developer.

6. Test-retest reliability information is reported far less frequently than alpha.

7. Factor analysis, which provides information about the structure of the scale, is used as another source of validity information for almost half of the scales.

8. More than half of the measures report convergent/divergent validity information with regard to significant positive and negative correlations in predictable directions with other measures. However, studies seem to be conducted in isolation so that rarely are two caring instruments used in the same study in order to establish criterion validity. In addition, the related measures selected by different authors to test relationships with their instrument rarely overlap.

9. The technique of using known groups or contrasting groups to establish the validity of caring instruments has rarely been used.

10. Discriminant validity defined as using the stringent multitrait-multimethod has not been reported in the literature on caring scale development.

11. Likewise, no studies were found which used a caring measure as predictive variable to predict a future score or event in a large-scale study.

Thus, it appears that even the most frequently used caring scale, the CARE-Q, has not as yet been used in sophisticated multivariate studies (to establish convergent/divergent validity, discriminant validity, and predictive validity), which would provide more convincing construct validity evidence. As a body of measurement tools, the strengths appear to lie in theoretical linkages to caring theories, conscious methods to establish content validity, factor analysis to assess structure, and relatively strong indicators of reliability (primarily internal consistency). Most of the instrument study designs have been descriptive, comparative, and/or correlational. At present, instrument development appears very isolated and fragmented. There are no studies that are using multiple caring tools and a matrix of other measures that should theoretically relate in positive and negative ways. Caring, apparently, is not being used as a predictor of future events or criteria.

ADDITIONAL MEASUREMENT ISSUES

RISKS OF RELIANCE ON SELF-REPORT MEASURES

Aside from the psychometric issues discussed above under the umbrella of construct validity, other serious measurement issues remain. Since most of the caring instruments involve self-report data, they run the risk of biased reporting that all self-report measures do. More studies need to be conducted which use triangulation of sources. While some studies have examined nurse caring ratings versus patient ratings, more studies need to be conducted using data from additional sources: perceptions of supervisors, clinical preceptors, and peers. Studies that compare self-report with observational data from objective trained observers would also be of interest. Triangulation of methods would also be helpful if, for example, comparisons could be made between paper and pencil measures and behavioral analysis of videotaped observations of nurses. There have been no studies to explore the relationships among the different types of caring purportedly assessed by the different scales. Caring abilities, caring efficacy, caring behaviors, and caring organizational climates could be studied concurrently with the same sample.

OTHER SAMPLING ISSUES

A seldom mentioned sampling issue is that the majority of the studies involve samples of nurses who are almost exclusively female. Lea and Watson (1996) suggest that male and female caregivers may have different conceptualizations of caring. A few investigators have been able to extend use of their scales so the focus was expanded to include other health care providers (e.g., Coates' 1999 sample of health care providers in a rehabilitation hospital; Swanson's 2000a consumer perceptions of health care professionals). Studies are needed to explore the caring measures with regard to basic demographic factors like gender, age, education, and experience. Often published studies using the caring measures neglect to describe how caring instruments relate to demographics. An international literature on assessing caring in different cultures is beginning (see CARE-Q matrix of

Swedish and Chinese studies and the Arthur et al., 1999 study of eleven different countries).

RESPONSE SET AND SOCIAL DESIRABILITY

The caring instrument developers have not systematically explored the issue of how response sets might affect the self-report caring instruments. Some test authors have taken the care to reduce response set bias by balancing the number of positively and negatively worded items in their Likert scales. A somewhat related issue is that of the positively skewed distributions of the caring test score distributions. How strong is the factor of social desirability? Perhaps the caring scales can be administered in concert with established measures of social desirability to begin to explore this potential bias. In addition, post-scale administration interviews might provide some insight into how respondents conceptualize and rate themselves on the scales.

SENSITIVITY

Since there have been very few studies which have explored change over time with regard to caring, the scales may possess sensitivity problems that have not yet been identified. "Sensitivity is the ability of an instrument to make discriminations of the fineness needed for the study" (Jacobson, 1997, p. 13). While it appears that a number of the caring tools have a sufficient degree of construct validity to begin to explore their effectiveness in outcome studies, at present very few research studies using caring as an outcome have been reported (Swanson, 1999). Steward and Archbold (1992) asserted: "In selecting an outcome measure for a study evaluating a nursing intervention, the criterion of sensitivity to change should predominate" (p. 477). Related to the positive skew of distributions in many of the caring scale studies, some of the caring instruments may have ceiling effects which will rule out their effectiveness for use in pre-post studies.

USABILITY

Usability or feasibility characteristics of the scales such as reading level, time to administer, and clarity of the directions have been reviewed with regard to most of the scales developed early on (see instrument descriptions presented earlier in this volume), but not with regard to the more recently developed ones. While potential users can estimate possible time to complete based on the number of items, more complete usability information for all of the caring instruments would be extremely useful for investigators trying to select the most appropriate scale for their research question and design.

SELECTION OF A CARING INSTRUMENT

The most basic question asked by potential users is whether the scale measures what one is attempting to assess about caring. Table 20.2 below is constructed as a guide to assist potential users in making initial choices based on measurement goals, scale type, respondents, and examples of applications.

Selecting a caring instrument for use in a research study is a complex task. "Multiple factors need to be taken into consideration in the decision-making process, such as the instrument's conceptual definition of caring, reliability and validity, length of time to administer, readability, and conceptual foundation" (Beck, 1999, pp. 29–30). Using the Table 20.2, a potential user can select a caring instrument or several instruments based on basic content and respondent characteristics, then move to explore the psychometric properties with regard to construct validity summarized in Table 20.1, and then, finally, examine the detailed instrument description and matrix summary (presented earlier in this volume) and the actual instrument. "Because few instruments have model histories, the evaluation of instruments always is a judgment call" (Jacobson, 1999, p. 16). In this volume (pp. 15–16) Jacobson outlined a series of important questions investigators should ask themselves when evaluating instruments.

Most of the instruments to assess caring were designed to assess nurse caring behaviors in a clinical setting from either the nurse and/or patient point of view. Duffy, Coates, and Hughes have designed instruments that are also appropriate to assess caring in nursing education. The Likert style instrument has been the primary format. While each scale author undoubtedly has much more information on the use of his/her instrument in different dissertations, program evaluations, and research studies, the use/applications listed above were primarily based on published information. Most of the instruments have been used in very limited ways (in addition to the primary instrument development studies). Very few have been used in educational or health care outcome studies as independent, dependent, or moderator variables.

TABLE 20.2 Basic Scale Information and Uses

CARING SCALE	CARING MEASUREMENT	SCALE TYPE	RESPONDENTS	EXAMPLES OF APPLICATIONS/USES
1. CARE-Q Larson, 1984	Caring behaviors	Q-Sort (Also, Swedish and Chinese versions.)	Patients Nurses Nursing students	Comparison of perceived importance of different nurse caring behaviors to patients versus nurses (See review of CARE-Q studies by Lea & Watson, 1996, p. 74; and review by Kyle, 1995, pp. 508–509.) Replications in Sweden (e.g., von Essen & Sjoden (1991a) and China (Holroyd et al, 1998).
2. CARE/SAT Larson & Ferketich, 1993	Satisfaction with caring behaviors	VAS	Patients	Limited to date.
3. CBI Wolf, 1986, 1994	Caring behaviors	Likert	Patients Nurses	Perceptions of nurse caring by post-operative patients (Swan, 1998)
4. CBA Cronin & Harrison, 1988	Caring behaviors	Likert	Patients	Perceptions of nurse caring by childbearing women (Manogin, Bechtel, & Rami, 2000); By HIV adults (Parsons, et al., 1993; Mullins, 1996); By institutionalized older adults (Marini, 1999); Comparison of antepartum and postpartum patients (Schultz, Bridgham, Smith, & Higgins, 1998)
5. CBNS Hinds, 1988	Caring behaviors	VAS	Patients	Limited to date.
6. PCB Horner, 1989, 1991	Caring behaviors	Likert	Patients Patient family members	Limited to date.

234

TABLE 20.2 *(continued)*

CARING SCALE	CARING MEASUREMENT	SCALE TYPE	RESPONDENTS	EXAMPLES OF APPLICATIONS/USES
7. CAS Nyberg, 1990	Caring attributes	Likert	Nurses	Limited to date.
8. CAI Nkongho, 1990	Caring abilities	Likert	Nurses Other professionals College students	Limited to date.
9. CBC McDaniel, 1990	Caring behaviors	Checklist	Trained observers	Limited to date.
10. CPC McDaniel, 1990	Response to caring behaviors	Likert	Patients	Limited to date.
11. CAT Duffy, 1992	Caring activities	Likert	Patients	Perceptions of nurse caring related to patient satisfaction (Duffy, 1992)
12. CAT-A Duffy, rev. 1993	Perceptions of managers' caring activities	Likert	Staff nurses	Staff nurses perceptions of administrator caring related to job satisfaction (Duffy, 1993)
13. CATedu Duffy, 2001	Perceptions of teaching/educational caring activities	Likert	Nursing students	Limited to date.
14. PGCS Hughes, 1993	Degree of caring of peer group climate	Likert	Student peer group in baccalaureate schools of nursing	Limited to date.

(continued)

TABLE 20.2 (*continued*)

CARING SCALE	CARING MEASUREMENT	SCALE TYPE	RESPONDENTS	EXAMPLES OF APPLICATIONS/USES
15. OCCQ Hughes, 1993	Degree of caring in organizational climate of baccalaureate nursing program	Likert	Nursing students	Limited to date.
16. CES Coates, 1995, 1997	Caring efficacy Caring efficacy of rated nurse/nursing student	Likert	Nurses/Nursing students Nursing supervisors/ Clinical preceptors Other health care providers	Program evaluation: nursing student outcomes (Coates, 1997) Effects of empowerment/caring training on health care providers' caring efficacy (Coates, 1999)
17. HCI Latham, 1988, 1996	Caring behaviors	Likert	Patients	Association between patient conditions and perceptions of nurse caring. Nurse caring contributes to patients' coping effectiveness. (Latham, 1996)
18. CDI Watson & Lea, 1997	Caring behaviors	Likert	Nurses	Limited to date.

TABLE 20.2 (*continued*)

CARING SCALE	CARING MEASUREMENT	SCALE TYPE	RESPONDENTS	EXAMPLES OF APPLICATIONS/USES
19. CAPSTI Arthur et al., 1998, 1999	Professional self-concept, technological influences, and caring attributes	Likert (translated into local languages of 11 countries)	Practicing nurses	Comparative international sample of practicing nurses in 11 countries. Studied caring attributes in relation to professional self-concept and technological influences (Arthur et al., 1999). Arthur reports two other international studies underway.
20. CPS Swanson, 2000	Practice relationship style: Compassionate healer and Competent practitioner	Likert	Nurses and other health care providers including physicians and midwives.	Assess caring as an intervention modality (sample of women who had experienced miscarriage) (Swanson 2000a & b)
21. MHCSNCI Sherwood & Shepherd, 2000	Satisfaction with caring	Likert	Patients	Program evaluation: Comparison of patient care units (Personal communication, Sherwood and Shepherd, 2000)

THE VIEW FROM EVIDENCE-BASED PRACTICE

Evidence-based practice has its foundations in England, but the concept is rapidly growing in acceptance in the U.S. as a way to gauge the quality of medical and nursing practice. However, evidence-based practice is currently a controversial topic in nursing. Barriers to moving nursing to an evidence-based practice discipline include insufficient research evidence, lack of time to find and evaluate the evidence, and perceived overreliance of medicine on the "gold standard" of randomized, double blind, controlled trials. Nevertheless, nurses cannot ignore the added press in the past few years to incorporate research utilization into their practice decisions because of technological changes that mean that consumers also have access to the latest research studies via the Internet and computer-based literature reviews. Reviews exploring the implications of evidence-based practice for nursing are increasing each year (English, 1998; Estabrooks, 1998; French, 1998; Giovannetti & O'Brien-Pallas, 1998; Ingersoll, 2000; King & Teo, 2000; Lang, 1999; McPheeters & Lohr, 1999; Nativio, 2000; Soukup, 2000).

An evidence-based approach puts a premium on certain kinds of research evidence, e.g., reviews and meta-analyses that present a body of research evidence, randomized, controlled trials, cohort studies, and case control studies. A lesser value is placed on descriptive, correlational, and qualitative studies (Gray, 1997; Greenhalgh, 1997; Guyatt et al., 1995).

The majority of quantitative research on measures of caring is primarily in the realm of descriptive, comparative, and correlational studies and is, therefore, lacking in terms of what is prized as the best evidence. Swanson (1999) reported she could only find three caring intervention studies that investigated the linkages between caring interventions and outcomes: Latham (1996) and Duffy (1992 and 1993). However, even these studies appear to employ correlational and comparative designs. Coates (1999) reported a significant pre-post gain in caring efficacy when evaluating a health care staff training intervention which emphasized enhancement of strategies of empowerment and caring; however, the study design was limited by the lack of a control group. There appear to be no reported outcome studies using robust experimental or quasi-experimental designs to assess caring-based interventions.

CONCLUSIONS AND RECOMMENDATIONS
FOR THE FUTURE

Psychometric Status of Instruments
to Measure Caring: Refinement

A variety of very creative approaches to assessing different domains of the concept of caring have been achieved through the work of a number of independent investigators. The instrument developers deserve credit for their struggles to achieve the difficult, but not impossible, task of developing credible measures of caring. Many of the researchers have pursued their work in the absence of external funding. The majority of the caring instruments, both first and second generation, have achieved a moderate degree of construct validity through theoretical linkages and conducting basic reliability and content validity testing.

Some measures would be enhanced by revisions based on principles of item analysis and factor analysis to clarify the structure of the instruments and to shore up scales based on too few items or subscales scoring lower in reliability. Almost all of the instruments would profit by utilizing large samples for the refinement process. Most of the scales are in dire need of anchoring their measures by correlational analysis with related and divergent measures, again with large samples. The technique of using known groups (samples predicted to be especially high or low on some aspect of caring) would help in this developmental process. All of these techniques will serve to refine and strengthen the psychometric properties of each instrument. So accumulation of evidence of construct validity may continue through its present course with a complex myriad of small studies. Some instruments will continue with the refinement process, and others may be truncated and not survive in the research literature.

ADVOCACY FOR INCREASED USE OF INSTRUMENTS TO MEASURE CARING

Continuance in building a web of evidence through small and diverse instrument development studies is not enough. A major leap has to be taken to advocate for more use of the scales in mainstream research and program evaluation studies in health care. There needs to be growth in the application of measures of caring in health care research to describe and define independent variables/caring interventions and to define dependent variables or outcomes. As the scales broaden their use and application, and researchers report reliability and validity information with a variety of samples, these efforts will serve to develop a substantial body of work sufficient to be described as achieving higher levels of construct validity.

There is a need to pursue funding for major research grants involving research questions around caring. Alternatively, perhaps some collaborative efforts may achieve these goals as well. The following are some suggestions for future research directions.

The first recommendation is consonant with one made by Valentine (1991) and supported by Lea and Watson (1996), i.e., the need for large multivariate studies. A large sample multitrait-multimethod study needs to be designed with a number of measures of caring included, as well as a large number of measures predicted to correlate positively and negatively with measures of caring. Work needs to be conducted with research designs, which triangulate sources of caring perceptions and methods of caring assessment.

Perhaps we are at a place now where we need to investigate how the various conceptions of caring—as ability, as behaviors, as efficacy beliefs, as organizational climates, etc.—relate to one another in nursing clinical arenas and in nursing educational enterprises. A causal modeling approach with a large sample might be extremely useful in beginning to explore how, or if, the various conceptions and measures of caring relate to each other. Swanson (1999) has begun some very important conceptual work in this area with her five levels of caring, and she has advocated that measurement work continue to address means to assess each level.

Caring constructs might be important as moderator variables. For example, there may be certain types of patients or clinical situations that are most responsive to caring interventions. Caring may be important as a moderator variable which enhances the effect of certain patient interventions or alternative care modalities. Patient situations involving high stress may make caring a more salient variable. Swanson (1999) suggested that qualitative findings about the context of caring should not be ignored.

Snyder et al. (2000) also supported the idea that quantitative data alone may not capture differences among nurses and situations. Qualitative data obtained through interviews may assist in explicating specific strategies nurses and other health care workers use to put into place caring orientations and climates. Coates (1999) found that staff training emphasizing caring resulted in significantly higher caring efficacy scores post-test; however, interviews with the trainees provided enriched descriptions of the nature of the changes. She found that in response to requests for vignettes about ways empowerment/caring training had affected them, health care providers could easily report: development of specific caring strategies that facilitated relationships with other staff members (and thereby, enhanced aspects of client care like enhanced case management across units); caring for the caregiver strategies they individually used to reduce stress and (and thereby made them more effective employees); and still other specific caring strategies that facilitated relationships with clients.

To support the well reasoned calls (Snyder, Brandt, & Tseng, 2000; Swanson, 1999) for more caring interventions in outcome studies, nurses need to be advocates for inclusion of measures of caring in large health care outcome studies with different patient populations. A majority of the caring instruments have not yet been utilized in studies to assess patient or student outcomes, despite the fact that a number of the instruments have demonstrated a sufficient level of construct validity to utilize them in more rigorous research designs. Swanson advocates " . . . a commitment to framing nursing intervention studies (caring actions) under the language of caring, hence providing a measurable and conceptually congruent framework to tie together the sound science underlying the practice of essential and professional nurse caring" (p. 56). Caring measures may be used as one of a number of outcome measures in traditional health care outcome studies as well as those focused on the effects of alternative care modalities.

The current literature represents a fragmented, non-integrated picture of numerous avenues to assess caring. To continue to concentrate only on instrument development without appropriate study in large-scale multivariate and outcome studies will ensure that the work will be disconnected from mainstream health care issues and research. For the body of work on caring measurement to have a significant and lasting impact on health care, caring measures with a moderate degree of construct validity need to be used in research studies to address important health care questions. Evidence-based nursing can be viewed as an opportunity to move forward using caring to define and assess the effects of nursing interventions and nursing education/training programs. It is time to move from the sidelines of health care research onto center stage. Appropriate *use* of the measures will mean that they will begin to fulfill their promise and create possibilities for exploring caring.

21

Postscript: Free Thoughts on Caring Theories and Instruments for Measuring Caring

Jean Watson

In reviewing the background of the development and evolution of the caring instruments, it may be helpful to summarize the relationship between extant caring theories and specific instruments. As noted in the discussions and the matrix cells, some instruments are guided formally by identified theories, some by multiple theories. Others are more empirically derived, while still others are reported to be atheoretical in origin. This section offers a general overview of the theoretical connections and origins of the diverse instruments, and seeks a more coherent view of the relationship between extant theories of caring and specific instruments. Please note that the categorizations are nonexclusive and overlapping.

A number of the instruments refer to the general caring theory literature and the conceptual aspects of caring without specific use of any given theory as a basis for formal instrumentation. I refer to these instruments as using *multiple concepts from extant caring theories* as broad guiding frameworks, as well as empirical strategies for item development. They include:

- CARE Q & CARE/SAT (Larson, 1984; Larson & Fertetich, 1993)
- Professional Caring Behavior (Horner, 1989)
- Client Perception of Caring Scale (McDaniel, 1990)
- Caring Dimensions Inventory (Watson & Lea, 1997)
- Caring Attributes Professional Self-Concept Technological Influence (Arthur, et al., 1999)

- Methodist Health Care System Nurse Caring Instrument (Shepherd & Sherwood, 2000)

Some instruments were developed from *formal identification and derivation of items from a specific caring theory or other relevant theory*. These theories and the instruments include:

- *Bandura's Social Learning Theory* from Social Psychology: Caring Efficacy Scale (Coates, 1995)
- *Howard's Humanistic Theory* from Psychology: Holistic Caring Inventory (Latham, 1988)
- *Mayeroff's Philosophy*: Caring Ability Inventory (Nkongho, 1990); Nyberg Caring Attributes Scale (Nyberg, 1990)
- *Paterson & Zderad's Humanistic Nursing Theory*: Caring Behavior of Nurses Scale (Hind, 1988)
- *Swanson's Caring Theory*: Caring Professional Scale (Swanson, 2000)

Understandably, it is interesting to me to discover that the most frequently reported theory in the caring instrument literature that informed the development of caring tools was *Watson's Theory of Caring* and *the 10 Carative Factors*. For example, the following instruments were based upon *Watson's Theory of Human Caring and/or the 10 Carative Factors*. Where used in nursing research, this instrument development and testing could be considered one form of empirical validation of Watson's theory, as well as development and validation of the instruments:

- Caring Behavior Inventory, CBI (Wolf, 1986)
- Caring Behavior Assessment, CBA (Cronin & Harrison, 1988)
- Nyberg Caring Attributes Scale, NCA (Nyberg, 1990)
- Caring Assessment Tools, CAT, CAT-admin, CAT-edu (Duffy, 1992, 2000)
- Caring Efficacy Scale, CES (Coates, 1995, 1997)

The following instruments can be characterized as primarily *empirically based* and they are largely atheoretical:

- Caring Dimensions Inventory (Watson & Lea, 1997)
- Caring Attributes Professional Self-Concept Technological Influence (Arthur et al., 1999)
- The CARE-Q (Larson, 1984)

Yet, even these most empirically derived caring instruments reportedly were informed, although indirectly, by early writings in the field of caring and by concepts embedded in those theoretical and general writings in the literature.

There are no hard conclusions that can be drawn about the relationship of caring theory and caring instruments, except to say that from the state of the science to date, the following seem to stand out as the *most theoretically grounded*

- *Mayeroff Caring Concepts & Philosophy*
  Nkongho Caring Ability Inventory
- *Paterson & Zderad Humanistic Nursing*
  Hinds Caring Behavior of Nurses Scale
- *Swanson Caring Theory*
  Swanson Caring Professional Scale
- *Watson's Caring Theory*
  Wolf Caring Behavior Inventory
  Cronin & Harrison Caring Behavior Nurses Scale
  Nyberg Caring Attributes Scale
  Duffy Caring Assessment Tool (CAT-admin & CAT-edu)
  Coates Caring Efficacy Scale

Those caring instruments that are most strongly *theoretically and empirically grounded* are:

- Cronin & Harrison's Caring Behavior Assessment
- Swanson's Caring Professional Scale

The instruments that are *most empirically grounded* based on studies with large samples are:

- Watson & Lea Caring Dimensions Inventory
- Arthur et al. Caring Attributes Professional Self-Concept Technological Influence
- Swanson Caring Professional Scale

The only instruments that focus on *organization and climate for caring* are:

- Hughes Peer Group Caring Interaction Scale
- Hughes Organizational Caring Climate Questionnaire

The most *educationally relevant* instruments are:

• Hughes Peer Group Scale
• Duffy Caring Assessment Tool (educational version)
• Coates Caring Efficacy Scale

Those instruments *most based and tested in clinical nursing practices* are:

• Larson CARE-Q
• Cronin & Harrison Caring Behavior Assessment
• Arthur et al. Caring Attributes Professional Self-Concept Technological Influence; Swanson Caring Professional Scale; and the latest Methodist Health Care System Nurse Caring Instrument
• Swanson Caring Professional Scale

The instruments most congruent with assessing caring *at the administrative level* are:

• Nyberg Caring Attributes Scale
• Duffy Caring Assessment Tool-admin
• Hughes Organizational Caring Climate Questionnaire

As one can readily see, several of the instruments fall into more than one category based on their origin and use. Other instruments have mixed use for students, clients, and nurses themselves, with many of the instruments used interchangeably for different audiences.

While various extant caring theories are acknowledged and used as a basis for the instruments in this book, there are other contemporary theories of caring upon which research is based that do not rely on empirical measures. For example, Figures 21.1 and 21.2 offer a closing visual view of extant caring theories and the various research and methodological traditions reflected by these contemporary theories, as well as a timeline for each instrument.

By way of closing remarks I offer the following reflections for the future of caring theory, instrumentation, and research. Rather than perpetuating a dualistic worldview that separates theory from practice and research, and isolates instrumentation and measurement from theoretical and conceptual relevance, different theories and measurement traditions need to begin to more systematically inform each other. The artificial dichotomy between qualitative and quantitative research and methods no longer can be sustained in such a complex world of clinical care. We have reached the paradoxical point that brings us both confusion and clarity in our

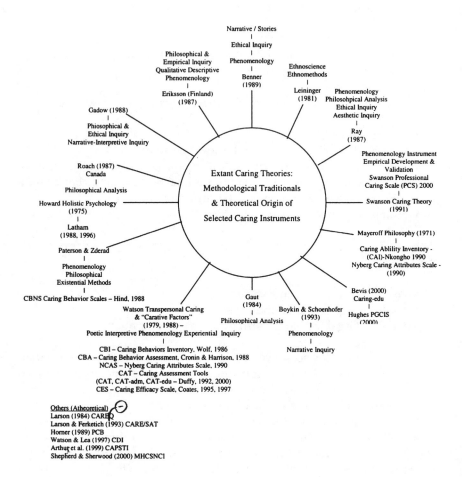

FIGURE 21.1 Extant caring theories: Methodological traditions and theoretical origin of selected caring instruments.

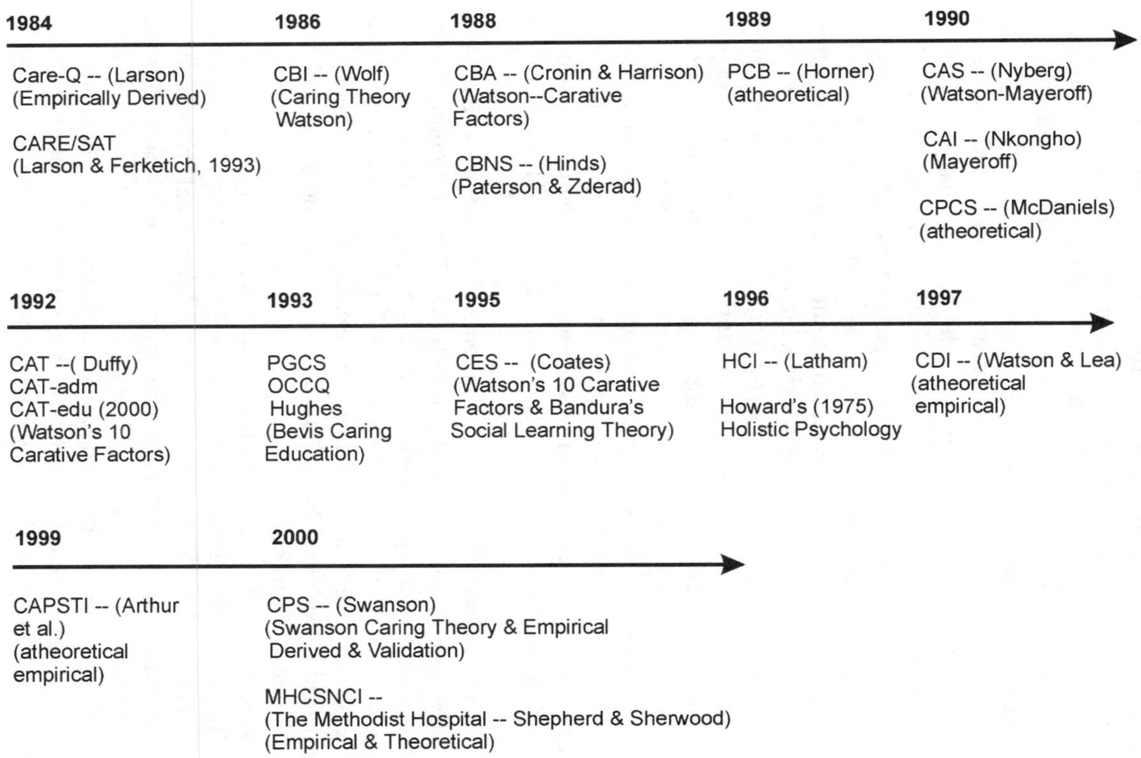

1984
Care-Q -- (Larson)
(Empirically Derived)

CARE/SAT
(Larson & Ferketich, 1993)

1986
CBI -- (Wolf)
(Caring Theory
Watson)

1988
CBA -- (Cronin & Harrison)
(Watson--Carative
Factors)

CBNS -- (Hinds)
(Paterson & Zderad)

1989
PCB -- (Horner)
(atheoretical)

1990
CAS -- (Nyberg)
(Watson-Mayeroff)

CAI -- (Nkongho)
(Mayeroff)

CPCS -- (McDaniels)
(atheoretical)

1992
CAT --(Duffy)
CAT-adm
CAT-edu (2000)
(Watson's 10
Carative Factors)

1993
PGCS
OCCQ
Hughes
(Bevis Caring
Education)

1995
CES -- (Coates)
(Watson's 10 Carative
Factors & Bandura's
Social Learning Theory)

1996
HCI -- (Latham)
Howard's (1975)
Holistic Psychology

1997
CDI -- (Watson & Lea)
(atheoretical
empirical)

1999
CAPSTI -- (Arthur
et al.)
(atheoretical
empirical)

2000
CPS -- (Swanson)
(Swanson Caring Theory & Empirical
Derived & Validation)

MHCSNCI --
(The Methodist Hospital -- Shepherd & Sherwood)
(Empirical & Theoretical)

FIGURE 21.2 Timeline of caring instrument development and theoretical origin.

phenomena and our methods. This paradoxical turn now invites an inclusion of all sources of data, both conventional and original sources. This is required if we are to move forward with meaningful forms of inquiry about the still largely unknown human phenomena of caring, healing processes, and outcomes. Therefore, multiple theories and multiple methods can begin to inform, enrich, and sharpen the focus of each other. Models of integration benefit from new developments; the different extant theories and research traditions, as well as new models emerging on the horizon can generate new and diverse research and data sources.

The relationship and interplay between caring theories and diverse approaches to measurement can lead to refinements, expansion, further explication, and validation of both current and emergent theories, as well as sophistication of instrumentation. The next generation of theory, research, methods, and measurements needs conceptual and operational space to develop and validate new grand theories, mini-theories, middle-range theories, and situation-specific theories, by exploring and uncovering old/new relationships and new understandings about the phenomenon of caring, between and among different populations and different human experiences. The next generation of caring research and instrument development needs freedom to pursue directions and multiple methods that explore the caring phenomenon in diverse practice domains, in educational caring curricula/pedagogies, and in administrative, environmental, structural, and system-organizational designs, thus revealing and bettering our knowledge of those caring practices operating at the ontological level where caring is lived.

The current cultural demands for evidence and outcomes invite and require a new generation of clinical research questions and multiple conceptual and operational approaches to assessment, evaluation, and measurement. Thus, the demand for theory-guided, theory-based, and theory-located contexts for evidence becomes even greater. Without a theoretical context for study, "evidence" becomes a hollow pursuit and does not build the discipline or the profession.

There is intellectual room and freedom in nursing science and all sciences at this new millennium turn to explore greater depths of construct validity for caring. This is an era to consider conceptual triangulation, theoretical-empirical triangulation, *and* instrument triangulation. This is a moment to dare to move between and beyond methods and dated research traditions. This is a time to entertain parallel and multisite studies, a period in history whereby we are called to reflect upon data and "evidence" from numbers, facts, texts, experience, self-reporting, observations, narrative, stories, interviews, dialogues, photos, videos, and perhaps even cyberspace, where physiological, technological, and ontological dimensions converge.

All of these challenges await nursing and all health professions. This work is embedded, grounded, and located in nursing science, but it is not just nursing—this work is by its very nature interdisciplinary, interprofessional and even transdisciplinary; it resides in that indeterminate zone of science and practice where all health practitioners and all patients ultimately live.

PARTING WORD

Finally, this work has just begun. The phenomenon of caring in nursing and health care awaits these new research traditions and new methodologies for assessing caring. In the meantime, the extant, contemporary caring instruments that have been developed await a new generation of replication, theoretical, conceptual, and empirical triangulation, and continuous approaches to validation and refinement. This is especially relevant with respect to new views of construct validity as well as the multiple meanings and approaches to assessing caring. Again, reminding ourselves that, in the end, all caring measurements are only one indicator of a human experience and ontological phenomena that offer at best some snapshots of a dynamic human dimension of *being* and *becoming*. Nevertheless, without incorporating caring into contemporary nursing and health sciences research, a core and vital aspect of nursing and health care will remain excluded and unknown.

References

Andrews, L. W., Daniels, P., & Hall, A. G. (1996). Nurse caring behaviors: Comparing five tools to define perceptions. *Ostomy/Wound Management, 42*(5), 28–37.

Arthur, D. (1995). Measurement of the professional self-concept of nurses: Developing a measurement instrument. *Nurse Education Today, 15,* 328–335.

Arthur, D., Pang, S., & Wong, T. (1998). Caring in context; Caring practices in a sample of Hong Kong nurses. *Contemporary Nurse, 7*(4), 198–204.

Authur, D., Pang, S., Wong, T., Alexander, M. F., Drury, J., et. al. (1999). Caring attributes, professional self-concept and technological influences in a sample of registered nurses in eleven countries. *International Journal of Nursing Studies, 36,* 387–396.

Arthur, D. (2001). *Personal Communication.*

Author. The Science of Caring UCSF. School of Nursing. (1988–2000).

Bandura, A. (1977). Self-efficacy: Toward a unified theory of behavioral change. *Psychological Review, 84,* 191–215.

Beck, C. T. (1999). Quantitative measurement of caring. *Journal of Advanced Nursing, 30*(1), 24–32.

Benner, P., & Wrubel, J. (1989). *The primacy of caring.* Menlo Park, CA: Addison-Wesley.

Bevis, E. O., & Watson, J. (2000). *Toward a caring curriculum,* Sudbury, MA: Jones & Bartlett.

Bowden, P. (1997). *Caring, Gender Sensitive Ethics,* London: Routledge.

Bork, R., Ereth, W., Fargo, B., & Kendall, B. (1983). Most important nurse caring behaviors as perceived by the oncology patient (unpublished manuscript). Montana State University School of Nursing.

Boykin, A., & Schoenhofer, S. (1993). *Nursing as caring.* New York: National League for Nursing.

Brody, J. (1988). Virtue ethics, caring and nursing. *Scholarly Journal for Nursing Practice, 2,* 87–101.

Brown, L. (1982). Behaviors of nurse perceived by hospitalized patients as indicators of care. Doctoral Dissertation, University of Colorado. *Dissertation Abstracts International, 42,* 436B. (University Microfilms #DA8209803.)

Brown, J., Kitson, A., & McKnight, T. (1992). *Challenges in Caring, Explorations in Nursing and Ethics.* London: Chapman and Hall.

Burns, N., & Grove, S. K. (2001). *The Practice of Nursing Research: Conduct, Critique, and Utilization* (4th ed.). Philadelphia: W. B. Saunders.

Campbell, D., & Fiske, D. (1959). Convergent and discriminant validation by the multitrait multi-method matrix. *Psychological Bulletin, 56,* 81–105.

Cavanaugh, S., & Simmons, P. (1997). Evaluation of a school climate for assessing affective objectives in health professional education. *Evaluation and the Health Professions, 20*(4), 455–478.

Coates, C. J. (1996). *Development of the Caring Efficacy Scale: Self-Report and Supervisor Versions.* Unpublished manuscript. Denver, CO: University of Colorado Health Sciences Center.

Coates, C. J. (1997). The caring efficacy scale: Nurses' self-reports of caring in practice settings. *Advanced Practice Nursing Quarterly, 3*(1), 53–59.

Coates, C. J. (1999). *Outcome Evaluation of Center for Healing and Renewal: Staff Professional Development Training.* Unpublished Manuscript. Boulder, Colorado: Boulder Community Hospital, Mapleton Rehabilitation Center.

Cronin, S., & Harrison, B. (1988). Importance of nurse caring behaviors as perceived by patients after myocardial infarction. *Heart and Lung, 17*(4), 374–380.

Duffy, J. (1990). The relationship between nurse caring behaviors and selected outcomes of care in hospitalized medical and/or surgical patients. Unpublished doctoral Dissertation. Catholic University of America, Washington, D.C.

Duffy, J. (1992). The impact of nurse caring on patient outcomes. In D. Gaut (Ed.), *The Presence of Caring in Nursing* (113–136). New York: NLN.

Duffy, J. (1993). Caring behaviors of nurse managers: Relationship to staff nurse satisfaction and retention. In D. Gaut (Ed.), *A Global Agenda for Caring* (365–378). New York: NLN.

Duffy, J. (2001). *Personal Communication.*

English, C. (1998). Evidence based nursing: Easier said than done. *Paediatric Nursing, 10*(5), 7–11.

Eriksson, K. (1987). Vardandets ide (The idea of caring). Stockholm: Alqvist & Wiksell Forlag AB.

Eriksson, K. (1994). Theories of caring as health. In D. Gaut & A. Boykin (Eds.), *Caring as healing: Renewal through hope* (3–18). New York: NLN.

Eriksson, K., & Lindstrom, U. (1999). A theory of science for caring science. *Hoito-tiede, 11*(6), 358–364.

Estabrooks, C. A. (1998). Will evidence-based nursing practice make practice perfect? *Canadian Journal of Nursing Research, 30*(1), 15–36.

Fagerstrom, L., & Engberg, I. B. (1998). Measuring the unmeasurable: A caring science perspective on patient classification. *Journal of Nursing Management, 6,* 165–172.

Fawcett, J. (1999). The state of nursing science: Hallmarks of the 20th and 21st centuries. *Nursing Science Quarterly, 12*(4), 311–318.

Fitzpatrick, J. J. (1995). Where has all the caring gone? *Applied Nursing Research, 8*(4), 155.

Ford, M. (1981). Nurse professionals and the caring process. Doctoral dissertation, University of Northern California. *Dissertation Abstracts International, 42,* 967B–968B. (University Microfilms No. 81 19278).

Frankel, R. (1994). Communicating with patients: Research shows it makes a difference. *MMI, Risk Management Resources, Inc.* Deerfield, IL: Risk Management Resources.

French, P. (1999). The development of evidence-based nursing. *Journal of Advanced Nursing, 29*(1), 72–78.

Fry, S. (1989). Towards a theory of nursing ethics. *Advances in Nursing Science, 11,* 9–22.

Gadow, S. A. (1988). Covenant without cure: Letting go and holding on in chronic illness. In J. Watson & M. Ray (Eds.), *The Ethics of Care, The Ethics of Cure.* New York: NLN.

Gadow, S. A. (1989). Clinical subjectivity. Advocacy with silent patients. *Nursing Clinics North America, 24,* 535–541.

Gaut, D. (1984). A theoretic description of caring as action. In M. Leininger (Ed.), *Care: The Essence of Nursing and Health* (pp. 27–44). Thorofare, NJ: Charles B. Slack.

Gay, S. (1999). Meeting cardiac patients' expectations of caring. *Dimensions of Critical Care Nursing, 18*(4), 46–50.

Giovannetti, P., & O'Brien-Pallas, L. L. (1998). From nursing data to information to evidence: are we prepared? *Canadian Journal of Nursing Research, 30*(1), 3–14.

Goodwin, L. D. (1997). Changing concepts of measurement validity. *Journal of Nursing Education, 36*(3), 102–107.

Gray, J. A. M. (1997). *Evidence-based health care: How to make health policy and management decisions.* New York: Churchill-Livingstone.

Green, J. L., & Stone, J. C. (1973). Teach me and I will be silent. A report of "Development and use of tools for curriculum evaluation." NIH, Nurse Project Training Grants NO. D 10 NU 00235-05.

Greenhalgh, J. (1997). *How to read a paper: The basics of evidence-based medicine.* London: BMJ Publishing Group.

Greenhalgh, J., Vanhanen, L., & Kyngas, H. (1998). Nursing care behaviors. *Journal of Advanced Nursing, 27,* 927–932.

Grobe, S. J., & Hughes, L. C. (1993). The conceptual validity of a taxonomy of nursing interventions. *Journal of Advanced Nursing, 21,* 652–658.

Guyatt, G. H., et al. (1995). User's guides to the medical literature IX. A method for grading health care recommendations. *JAMA, 274,* 1800–18004.

Halldorsdottir, S. (1999). The effects of uncaring. *Reflections.* International Sigma Theta Tau, Fourth Quarter, 28–30.

Harrison, E. (1995). Nurse caring and the new health care paradigm. *Journal of Nursing Care Quality, 9*(4), 14–23.

Henry, D. M. M. (1975). Nurse behaviors perceived by patients as indicators of caring. Doctoral dissertation, Catholic University. *Dissertation Abstracts International, 36*(02 652B). University Microfilms NO. 75 16:229.

Hinds, P. S. (1985). An investigation of the relationship between adolescent hopefulness, caring behaviors of nurses, and adolescent health care outcomes. *Dissertation Abstracts International, 4012.* University Microfilms No. 8522813.

Hinds, P. (1988). The relationship of nurses' caring behaviors with hopefulness and health care outcomes in adolescents. *Archives of Psychiatric Nursing, 2*(1), 21–29.

Hinshaw, A., & Atwood, J. (1982). A patient satisfaction instrument: Precision by replication. *Nursing Research, 31,* 170–175.

Hinshaw, A. S. (2000). Nursing knowledge for the 21st century: Opportunities and challenges. *Journal of Nursing Scholarship, 32*(2), 117–123.

Holroyd, E., Yue-kuen, C., Sau-wai, C., Fund-sham, L., & Wai-wan, W. (1998). A Chinese cultural perspective of nursing care behaviours in an acute setting. *Journal of Advanced Nursing, 28*(6), 1289–1294.

Howard, J. (1975). Humanization and dehumanization of health care: A conceptual view. In J. Howard & A. Strauss (Eds.), *Humanizing health care* (57–102). New York: John Wiley. (In Latham, 1996)

Huber, D. I., Maas, M., McCloskey, J., Scherb, C. A., Goode, C. J., & Watson, C. (2000). Evaluating nursing administration instruments. *Journal of Nursing Administration, 30*(5), 251–272.

Huggins, K., Gandy, W., & Kohut, C. (1993). Emergency department patient perceptions of nurse caring behaviors. *Heart and Lung, 22*(4), 356–364.

Hughes, L. A. (1992). Faculty-student interactions and the student-perceived climate for caring. *ANS, 14*(3), 60–71.

Hughes, L. (1993). Peer group interactions and the student-perceived climate for caring. *Journal of Nursing Education, 32*(2), 78–83.

Hughes, L. C. (1998). Development of an instrument to measure caring peer group interactions. *Journal of Nursing Education, 37*(5), 202–207.

Hughes, L. (2001). Personal Communication. Unpublished Manuscript.

Hulela, E. B., Akinsola, H. A., & Sekoni, N. M. (2000). The observed nurses caring behavior in a referral hospital in Botswana. *West African Journal of Nursing, 11*(1), 1–6.

Ingersoll, G. L. (2000). Evidence-based nursing: What it is and what it isn't. *Nursing Outlook, 48*(4), 151–152.

Jacobson, S. F. (1997). Evaluating instruments for use in clinical nursing research. In M. Frank-Stromborg & S. J. Olsen (Eds.), *Instruments for clinical health care research*, 00.3–19. Sudbury, MA: Jones and Bartlett.

Kiesler, D. J. (1987). *Manual for the Impact of Message Inventory: Research Edition.* Palo Alto, CA: Consulting Psychologists Press. (In Latham, 1996).

Kim, H. S. (1996). Challenges of new perspectives. *Nursing Knowledge Impact Conference.* Boston: Boston College School of Nursing.

King, K. M., & Teo, K. K. (2000). Integrating clinical quality improvement strategies with nursing research. *Western Journal of Nursing Research, 22*(5), 596–608.

Komorita, N., Koehring, K., & Hirchert, P. (1991). Perceptions of caring by nurse educators. *Journal of Nursing Education, 30*(1), 23–29.

Kuhse, H. (1993). Caring is not enough: Reflections on a nursing ethics of care. *Australian Journal of Advanced Nursing, 11*, 32–41.

Kyle, T. V. (1995). The concept of caring: A review of the literature. *Journal of Advanced Nursing, 21*, 506–514.

LaMonica, E. (1981). Construct validity of an empathy instrument. *Research in Nursing and Health, 4*, 389–400.

Lang, N. M. (1999). Discipline-based approaches to evidence-based practice: A view from nursing. *Joint Commission Journal on Quality Improvement, 25*(10), 539–544.

Larson, P. (1984). Important nurse caring behaviors perceived by patients with cancer. *Oncology Nursing Forum, 11*, 46–50.

Larson, P. (1986). Cancer nurses' perceptions of caring. *Cancer Nursing, 9*(2), 86–91.

Larson, P. (1987). Comparison of cancer patients' and professional nurses' perceptions of important nurse caring behaviors. *Heart and Lung, 16*(2), 187–193.

Larson, P., & Ferketich, S. (1993). Patients' satisfaction with nurses' caring during
hospitalization. *Western Journal of Nursing Research, 15*(6), 690–707.

Latham, C. P. (1988). *Measurement of Caring in Recipient-Provider Interactions.* Proceedings of the Second Annual Measurement of Clinical and Educational Nursing
Outcomes Conference. Sago, CA.

Latham, C. P. (1996). Predictors of patient outcomes following interaction with
nurses. *Western Journal of Nursing Research, 18*(5), 548–564.

Lea, A., & Watson, R. (1996). Caring research and concepts: A selected review of
the literature. *Journal of Clinical Nursing, 5,* 71–77.

Lea, A., Watson, R., & Deary, I. J. (1998). Caring in nursing: A multivariate analysis.
Journal of Advanced Nursing, 28(3), 662–671.

Lea, A., & Watson, R. (1999). Research in brief. Perceptions of caring among nurses:
The relationship to clinical area. *Journal of Clinical Nursing, 8*(5), 617–618.

Leininger, M. M. (1981). The phenomenon of caring: Importance, research questions and theoretical considerations. In M. M. Leininger (Ed.), *Caring: An essential
human need* (pp. 2–15). Thorofare, NJ: Slack.

Lindstrom, U., & Eriksson, K. (1999). The fundamental idea of quality assurance.
International Journal for Human Caring, 3(3), 21–27.

Mangold, A. (1991). Senior nursing students' & professional nurses' perceptions
of effective caring behaviors: A comparative study. *Journal of Nursing Education,
30*(3), 134–139.

Manogin, T. W., Bechtel, G. A., & Rami, J. S. (2000). Caring behaviors by nurses:
Women's perceptions during childbirth. *JOGNN, 29*(2), 153–157.

Marini, B. (1999). Institutionalized older adults' perceptions of nurse caring behaviors. *Journal of Gerontological Nursing, 25*(5), 11–16.

Mayer, D. (1986). Cancer patients' and families' perceptions of nurse caring behaviors. *Topics in Clinical Nursing, 8*(2), 63–69.

Mayer, D. (1987). Oncology nurses' vs. cancer patients' perceptions of nurse caring
behaviors: A replication study. *Oncology Nursing Forum, 14*(3), 48–52.

Mayeroff, M. (1971). *On caring.* New York: Harper & Row.

McCance, T., McKenna, H., & Boore, J. (1997). Caring: Dealing with a difficult
concept. *International Journal of Nursing Studies, 34*(4), 241–248.

McDaniel, A. (1990). The caring process in nursing: Two instruments for measuring
caring behaviors. In O. Strickland & C. Waltz (Eds.), *Measurements of Nursing
Outcomes* (pp. 17–27). New York: Springer.

McPheeters, M., & Lohr, K. N. (1999). Evidence practice and nursing: Commentary.
Outcomes Management for Nursing Practice, 3(3), 99–101.

Morse, J. M., Bottorff, J., Neander, W., & Solberg, S. (1991). Comparative analysis
of conceptualizations and theories of caring. *Image: Journal of Nursing Scholarship,
23,* 119–127.

Mullins, I. L. (1996). Nurse caring behaviors for persons with Acquired Immunodeficiency Syndrome/Human Immunodeficiency Virus. *Applied Nursing Research,
9*(1), 18–23.

Nativio, D. G. (2000). Guidelines for evidence-based clinical practice. *Nursing Outlook, 48*(2), 58–59.

Newman, M. A., Sime, A. M., & Corcoran-Perry, S. A. (1991). The focus of the discipline of nursing. *ANS, 14*(1), 1–6.

Nkongho, N. (1990). The Caring Ability Inventory. In O. Strickland & C. Waltz (Eds.), *Measurement of Nursing Outcomes* (pp. 3–16). New York: Springer.

Noddings, N. (1994). *Caring: A feminine approach to ethics and moral development.* Berkeley: University of California.

Nunnally, J., & Bernstein, I. (1994). *Psychometric Theory.* New York: McGraw-Hill.

Nyberg, J. (1990). The effects of care and economics on nursing practice. *Journal of Nursing Administration, 20*(5), 13–18.

Parsons, E., Kee, C., & Gray, P. (1993). Perioperative nursing caring behaviors. *AORN Journal, 57*(5), 1106–1114.

Paterson, J. G., & Zderad, L. T. (1976). *Humanistic nursing.* New York: Wiley.

Phillips, P. (1993). A deconstruction of caring. *Journal of Advanced Nursing, 18,* 1554–1558.

Polit, D. F., & Hungler, B. P. (1999). *Nursing Research: Principles and methods* 6th ed. Philadelphia: Lippincott.

Ray, M. A. (1987). Technological caring: A new model in critical care. *Dimensions Critical Care Nursing, 6*(3), 166–173.

Roach, M. S. (1987). *The human act of caring: A blueprint for health professions.* Toronto, Canada: Canadian Hospital Association.

Robinson, J. P., Shaver, P. R., & Wrightsman, L. S. (1991). Criteria for scale selection and evaluation. In J. P. Robinson, P. R. Shaver, & L. S. Wrightsmans (Eds.), *Measures of personality and social psychological attitudes* (pp. 1–16). San Diego: Academic Press.

Rogers, M. E. (1970). *An introduction to the theoretical basis of nursing.* Philadelphia: Davis.

Rosenthal, K. (1992). Coronary care patients' and nurses' perceptions of important nurse caring behaviors. *Heart and Lung, 21*(6), 536–539.

Schultz, A. A., Bridgham, C., Smith, M. E., & Higgins, D. (1998). Perceptions of Caring: Comparison of antepartum and postpartum patients. *Clinical Nursing Research, 7,* 363–378.

Shepherd, M. L., Sherwood, G. D., Rude, M. B., & Eriksen, L. R. (2001). Methodist Health Care System Development of Nursing Caring Instrument. *Personal Communication.* Unpublished Manuscript.

Simmons, P. R., & Cavanaugh, S. H. (2000). Relationships among student and graduate caring ability and professional school climate. *Journal of Professional Nursing, 16*(2), 76–83.

Smith, M., & Reeder, F. (1998). Clinical outcomes research and Rogerian science: Strange or emergent bedfellows? *Visions, 6*(1), 27–38.

Smith, M. (1999). Caring and the Science of Unitary Human Beings. *Advances in Nursing Science, 21*(4), 14–28.

Smith, M. K., & Sullivan, J. M. (1997). Nurses' and patients' perceptions of most important caring behaviors in a long-term care setting. *Geriatric Nursing, 18,* 70–73.

Snyder, M., Brandt, C. L., & Tseng, Y. (2000). Measuring intervention outcomes: Impact of nurse characteristics. *International Journal for Human Caring*, Spring, 36–42.

Soukup, S. M. (2000). The Center for Advanced Nursing Practice evidence-based practice model: Promoting the scholarship of practice. *Nursing Clinics of North America*, 35(2), 301–309.

Stanfield, M. H. (1992). Watson's caring theory and instrument development. *Dissertation Abstracts International*, 52(8). Order NO. DA. 9203096: 4128-B.

Stewart, B. J., & Archbold, P. G. (1992). Focus on psychometrics: Nursing intervention studies require outcomes measures that are sensitive to change: Part one. *Research in Nursing and Health*, 15, 477–481.

Stewart, B. J., & Archbold, P. G. (1997). A new look for measurement validity. Guest Editorial. *Journal of Nursing Education*, 36(3), 99–101.

Stockdale, M., & Warelow, P. J. (2000). Is the complexity of care a paradox? *Journal of Advanced Nursing*, 31(5), 1258–1264.

Strickland, O. L., & Waltz, C. F. (1990). *Measurement of Nursing Outcomes, Vol. Four.* New York: Springer.

Swan, B. A. (1998). Postoperative nursing care contributions to symptom distress and functional status after ambulatory surgery. *MEDSURG Nursing*, 7(3), 148–151, 154–158.

Swanson, K. (1991). Empirical development of a middle-range theory of caring. *Nursing Research*, 40, 161–166.

Swanson, K. (1999). What is known about caring in nursing science. In A. S. Hinshaw, S. Fleetham, & J. Shaver (Eds.), *Handbook of Clinical Nursing Research* (pp. 31–60). Thousand Oaks, CA: Sage.

Swanson, K. (2000a). Predicting depressive symptoms after miscarriage: A path analysis based on the Lazarus paradigm. *Journal of Women's Health & Gender-Based Medicine*, 9(2), 2000, 191–206.

Swanson, K. (2000b). A program of research on caring. In M. E. Parker (Ed.), *Nursing Theories and Nursing Practice*. Philadelphia: F. A. Davis.

Tresolini, C. P., & Pew-Fetzer Task Force. (1994). *Health Professions Education and Relationship Centered Care*. San Francisco: Pew Health Professions Commission.

Valentine, K. (1991). Nurse-patient caring: Challenging our conventional wisdom. In D. A. Gaut & M. M. Leininger (Eds.), *Caring: The compassionate healer* (pp. 99–113). New York: National League for Nursing.

von Essen, L., & Sjoden, P. (1991a). The importance of nurse caring behaviors as perceived by Swedish Hospital Patients and nursing staff. *International Journal of Nursing Studies*, 28(3), 267–281.

von Essen, L., & Sjoden, P. (1991b). Patient and staff perceptions of caring: Review and replication. *Journal of Advanced Nursing*, 16(11), 1363–1374.

von Essen, L., & Sjoden, P. (1993). Perceived importance of caring behaviors to Swedish Psychiatric inpatients and staff with comparisons to somatically-ill samples. *Research in Nursing and Health*, 16, 293–303.

Walsh, M. (1999). Nurses and nurse practitioners 1: Priorities in care. *Nursing Standard*, 13(24), 38–42.

Waltz, C. R. Strickland, O. L., & Lenz, E. R. (1984). *Measurement in Nursing Research.* Philadelphia: F. A. Davis.

Waltz, C. F., Strickland, O. L., & Lenz, E. R. (1991). *Measurement in Nursing Research,* 2nd ed. Philadelphia: Davis.

Watson, J. (1979). *Nursing: The philosophy and science of caring.* Boston: Little, Brown. Reprinted (1985). Boulder: Colorado Associated University Press.

Watson, J. (1988). *Nursing: Human Science and Human Care. A Theory of Nursing.* New York: National League for Nursing.

Watson, J. (1990). Caring knowledge and informed moral passion. *Advances in Nursing Science, 13,* 15–24.

Watson, J., & Phillips, S. (1992). A call for educational reform: Colorado nursing doctorate model as exemplar. *Nursing Outlook, 40*(1), 20–26.

Watson, J., & Smith, M. (2000). Re-visioning caring science and Rogerian science of unitary human beings. Paper presented at Boston Knowledge Development Conference. Boston: Boston College School of Nursing.

Watson, R., & Lea, A. (1997). The caring dimensions inventory. (CDI), Content validity, reliability, and scaling. *Journal of Advanced Nursing, 25,* 87–94.

Watson, R., Deary, I. J., & Lea, A. (1999). A longitudinal study into the perceptions of caring among nursing students using multivariate analysis of the Caring Dimension Inventory. *Journal of Advanced Nursing, 30,* 1080–1089.

Widmark-Petersson, V., von Essen, L., & Sjoden, P. (1998). Perceptions of caring: Patients' and staff's associations to CARE-Q behaviors. *Journal of Psychosocial Oncology, 16*(1), 75–79.

Widmark-Petersson, V., von Essen, L., & Sjoden, P. (2000). Perceptions of caring among patients with cancer and their staff: differences and disagreements. *Cancer Nursing, 23*(1), 32–39.

Williams, S. A. (1998). Quality and care: Patients' perceptions. *Journal Nursing Care Quality, 12*(6), 18–25.

Wolf, Z. R. (1986). The caring concept and nurse identified caring behaviors. *Topics in Clinical Nursing, 8*(2), 84–93.

Wolf, Z. R., Giardino, E. R., Osborne, P. A., & Ambrose, M. S. (1994). Dimensions of nurse caring. *Image: Journal of Nursing Scholarship, 26*(2), 107–111.

Wolf, Z. R., Colahan, M., Costello, A., Warwick, F., Ambrose, M. S., & Giardino, E. R. (1998). Research utilization: Relationship between nurse caring and patient satisfaction. *MEDSURG Nursing, 7*(2), 99–105.

APPENDIX

Master Matrix Blueprint
for All Instruments
for Measuring Caring

Master Matrix Blueprint for All Instruments for Measuring Caring

Instrument	Author Contact Address	Publication Citation Source	Developed to Measure	Instrument Description	Participants	Reported Validity/ Reliability	Conceptual/ Theoretical Basis of Measurement	Latest Citation in Nursing Literature
Caring Assessment Instrument (CARE-Q) 1984	Patricia Larson, RN, DNS (Retired from) Univ. of California, San Francisco (UCSF) School of Nursing Department of Physiology Nursing Box 0610 N 611Y San Francisco, CA 94143-0610 *pattakw@ msn.com*	Larson, P. (1984). Important nurse caring behaviors perceived by patients with cancer. *Oncology Nursing Forum, 11*(6), 46–50.	Perceptions of nurse caring behaviors	Q-sort 50 cards into 7 piles/7 point scale to prioritize perceptions of nurse caring behaviors Noted to be confusing, ambiguous to administer, and time-consuming; but most commonly used, both nationally and internationally	Patients (oncology) n = 57	Expert panel test-retest Content and face validity	General references to nursing theories of caring A priori development Guided by care needs of cancer patients	Chinese version of Care-Q 1998 Holroyd, E., Yue-kuen, C., Sau-wai, C., Fungshan, L., 7 Wai-wan, W. (1998) A Chinese cultural perspective of nursing care behaviors in an acute setting. *Joural of Advanced Nursing, 28*(6), 1289–1294.

Master Matrix Blueprint for All Instruments for Measuring Caring *(continued)*

Instrument	Author Contact Address	Publication Citation Source	Developed to Measure	Instrument Description	Participants	Reported Validity/ Reliability	Conceptual/ Theoretical Basis of Measurement	Latest Citation in Nursing Literature
								Hulela, E. B., Akinsola, H. A. & Sekoni, N. M. (2000). The observed nurses caring behavior in a referral hospital in Botswana. *West African Journal of Nursing, 11*(1), 1–6.

(continued)

Master Matrix Blueprint for All Instruments for Measuring Caring *(continued)*

Instrument	Author Contact Address	Publication Citation Source	Developed to Measure	Instrument Description	Participants	Reported Validity/ Reliability	Conceptual/ Theoretical Basis of Measurement	Latest Citation in Nursing Literature
CARE-Q	Larson, P. (UCSF)	Larson, P. (1986). Cancer nurses' perceptions of caring. *Cancer Nursing, 9*(2), 86–91.	Perceptions of nurse caring behaviors	Q-Sort	Nurses (oncology) n = 57	Extension of Larson, 1984 See Larson, 1984	ditto	ditto

Master Matrix Blueprint for All Instruments for Measuring Caring *(continued)*

Instrument	Author Contact Address	Publication Citation Source	Developed to Measure	Instrument Description	Participants	Reported Validity/ Reliability	Conceptual/ Theoretical Basis of Measurement	Latest Citation in Nursing Literature
CARE-Q	Larson, P. (UCSF)	Larson, P. (1987). Comparison of cancer patients and professional nurses' perceptions of important nurse caring behaviors. *Heart & Lung, 16*(2), 187–192.	Identifies nurse caring behaviors	Q-Sort	Nurses (oncology) n = 57 Patients (oncology) n = 57	See Larson, 1984	ditto	ditto

(continued)

Master Matrix Blueprint for All Instruments for Measuring Caring *(continued)*

Instrument	Author Contact Address	Publication Citation Source	Developed to Measure	Instrument Description	Participants	Reported Validity/ Reliability	Conceptual/ Theoretical Basis of Measurement	Latest Citation in Nursing Literature
CARE-Q Replication study and use	Mayer, D. RN, PhD, Clinical specialist, Mass. General Hospital	Mayer (1987). Oncology nurses vs. cancer patients' perceptions of nurse caring behaviors: A replication study. *Oncology Nursing Forum, 14*(3), 48–52.	Evaluates nurse caring behaviors	Q-Sort	Nurses (oncology) n = 28 Patients (oncology) n = 54	Content and face validity Test-retest reliability (refers to Larson, 1984 original testing)	Replication of instrument; plus extension of conceptual foundation of original Larson (1984) version of Care-Q	ditto

Master Matrix Blueprint for All Instruments for Measuring Caring *(continued)*

Instrument	Author Contact Address	Publication Citation Source	Developed to Measure	Instrument Description	Participants	Reported Validity/ Reliability	Conceptual/ Theoretical Basis of Measurement	Latest Citation in Nursing Literature
CARE-Q	Nori Komorita, PhD, RN Kathleen Doehring, MS, RN Phyllis Hirchert, MS, RN Urbana Regional Program, College of Nursing, U. of Illinois, Urbana	Komorita, N., Doehring, K., Hirchert, P. (1991). Perceptions of caring by nurse educators. *Journal of Nursing Education,* 30(1), 23–29.	Nurse educators' perceptions of caring behaviors	Q-Sort	Nurse Educators n = 110	Refers to Larson's original work (1984)	Caring in relation to nursing education No new reliability or validity reported for nursing educational use	ditto

(continued)

266

Master Matrix Blueprint for All Instruments for Measuring Caring *(continued)*

Instrument	Author Contact Address	Publication Citation Source	Developed to Measure	Instrument Description	Participants	Reported Validity/ Reliability	Conceptual/ Theoretical Basis of Measurement	Latest Citation in Nursing Literature
CARE-Q	Antonia Mangold MSN, RN Oncology Clinical Staff Nurse Thomas Jefferson University Hospital, Philadelphia	Manford, A. (1991). Senior nursing students' & Professional Nurses' Perceptions of Effective Caring Behaviors: A Comparative Study. *Journal of Nursing Education, 30(3)*, 134–139.	Identifies and compares nursing students and RNs' perception of caring behaviors	Q-Sort	Nursing Students n = 30	See Larson (1984) Original citation for test-retest reliability	Larson's original conceptual basis; plus informed by Watson's 10 carative factors	ditto

Master Matrix Blueprint for All Instruments for Measuring Caring *(continued)*

Instrument	Author Contact Address	Publication Citation Source	Developed to Measure	Instrument Description	Participants	Reported Validity/ Reliability	Conceptual/ Theoretical Basis of Measurement	Latest Citation in Nursing Literature
CARE-Q	Louise von Essen MS, Psychology; Per-Olow Sjoden, PhD Center for Caring Sciences, Uppsala University Akademiska Hospital, S-751 85 Uppsala, SWEDEN *Louise-von.essen@cc-s.uu.se*	Von Essen & Sjoden (1991a). The importance of nurse caring behaviors as perceived by Swedish hospital patients and nursing staff. *International Journal of Nursing Studies, 28(3),* 267–281.	Perceived caring behaviors by nurses and patients	Q-Sort **(International Swedish Version)**	Oncology, General Surgery Orthodpedic patients n = 81 Nurses n = 105	No reliability or validity reported for Swedish version Refers to information reported by Larson (1981, 1984)	Affective components of care and a caring relationship	Larsson, G. Petersson, V. W., Lampic, C., von Essen, L., Sjoden, P. (1998). Cancer patient and staff rating of the importance of caring behaviors and their relation to patient anxiety and depression. *Journal of Advanced Nursing, 27,* 855–864.

(continued)

Master Matrix Blueprint for All Instruments for Measuring Caring *(continued)*

Instrument	Author Contact Address	Publication Citation Source	Developed to Measure	Instrument Description	Participants	Reported Validity/ Reliability	Conceptual/ Theoretical Basis of Measurement	Latest Citation in Nursing Literature
								Widmark-Petersson, V., von Essen, L. & Sjoden, P. (1998). Perceptions of caring: patients and staff's association to CARE-Q behaviours. *Journal of Psychosocial Oncology, 16(1)*, 75–96.

Master Matrix Blueprint for All Instruments for Measuring Caring *(continued)*

Instrument	Author Contact Address	Publication Citation Source	Developed to Measure	Instrument Description	Participants	Reported Validity/ Reliability	Conceptual/ Theoretical Basis of Measurement	Latest Citation in Nursing Literature
CARE-Q	Louise von Essen & Per-Olow Sjoden, Uppsala University SWEDEN (see above)	von Essen, & Sjoden, P. (1991). Patient & Staff Perceptions of Caring: Review and Replication. *Journal of Advanced Nursing, 16*(11), 1363–1374.	Perceived caring behaviors by nurses and patients (Swedish population)	**International Version** Q-Sort of same items of 7 point scale (Swedish version) Replication of 1991 study Questionnaires with items of Q-Sort	Nurses n = 73 Medical patients n = 86	See von Essen & Sjoden (1991a)		Widmark-Petersson, V. von Essen, L. & Sjoden, P. (2000). Perceptions of caring among patients with cancer and their staff: differences and disagreements. *Cancer Nursing, 23*(1), 32–39.

(continued)

Master Matrix Blueprint for All Instruments for Measuring Caring   *(continued)*

Instrument	Author Contact Address	Publication Citation Source	Developed to Measure	Instrument Description	Participants	Reported Validity/ Reliability	Conceptual/ Theoretical Basis of Measurement	Latest Citation in Nursing Literature
CARE-Q	Kathryn Rosenthal, MS, RN University of Colorado	Rosenthal, K. (1992). Coronary care patients' and nurses' perceptions of important nurse caring behaviors. *Heart & Lung, 21*(6), 536–539.	Examines the relationship of patient-perceived and nurse-perceived caring behaviors	Q-Sort	Coronary nurses n = 30 Coronary Patients n = 30	See Larson (1984, 1987)	General nursing caring literature(Larson, 1984, 1987 for tool) Watson et al. included in background of study	None to date

Master Matrix Blueprint for All Instruments for Measuring Caring *(continued)*

Instrument	Author Contact Address	Publication Citation Source	Developed to Measure	Instrument Description	Participants	Reported Validity/ Reliability	Conceptual/ Theoretical Basis of Measurement	Latest Citation in Nursing Literature
CARE-Q	Louise von Essen, Per-Olow Sjoden, Uppsala University, Sweden (see above)	Von Essen, L. & Sjoden, P. (1993). Perceived importance of caring behaviors to Swedish psychiatric inpatients and staff with comparisons to somatically-ill samples. *Research in Nursing & Health, 16,* 293–303.	Nurse caring behaviors as perceived by psychiatric patients with comparison to somatically-ill patients	Q-Sort comparative study with different patient populations **International Swedish version of tool modified** for psychiatric patients (used free response format)	Mental Health nurses n = 63 (Psychiatric nurses, RNs, and students) Mental health patients n = 61	Discussion of difficulty with Q-Sort Found to be unreliable due to forced distribution Discusses internal consistency using a free response format Content validity addressed	See above Perception of Caring relationship and caring behaviors	Larsson, G., Petersson, V. W., Lampic, C., von Essen, L., Sjoden, P. (1998). Cancer patient and staff rating of the importance of caring behaviors and their relation to patient anxiety and depression. *Journal of Advanced Nursing, 27,* 855–864.

(continued)

Master Matrix Blueprint for All Instruments for Measuring Caring *(continued)*

Instrument	Author Contact Address	Publication Citation Source	Developed to Measure	Instrument Description	Participants	Reported Validity/ Reliability	Conceptual/ Theoretical Basis of Measurement	Latest Citation in Nursing Literature
								Widmark-Petersson, V., von Essen, L., & Sjoden, P. (2000). Perceptions of caring among patients with cancer and their staff: differences and disagreements. *Cancer Nursing, 23*(1), 32–39.

273

Master Matrix Blueprint for All Instruments for Measuring Caring *(continued)*

Instrument	Author Contact Address	Publication Citation Source	Developed to Measure	Instrument Description	Participants	Reported Validity/ Reliability	Conceptual/ Theoretical Basis of Measurement	Latest Citation in Nursing Literature
CARE-Q	Margaret K. Smith, RN, MSN Assistant Nurse Manager, Nursing Home Care Unit VA Palo Alto Health Care System, Menlo Park, CA	Smith, M. (1997). Nurses' and patients' perceptions of most important caring behaviors in a long-term care setting. *Geriatric Nursing, 18*(2), 70–73.	Compare rankings of caring behaviors as perceived by patients and nurses	50 items with 6 sub-scales Q-Sort	n = 12 men; 2 women patients; n = 15 RNs from nursing home care unit at Veterans Affairs Medical Center	Reliability or validity not addressed	No theoretical/conceptual model mentioned	ditto

(continued)

Master Matrix Blueprint for All Instruments for Measuring Caring *(continued)*

Instrument	Author Contact Address	Publication Citation Source	Developed to Measure	Instrument Description	Participants	Reported Validity/ Reliability	Conceptual/ Theoretical Basis of Measurement	Latest Citation in Nursing Literature
CARE-Q	Greenhalgh, J., Vanha-nen, L., & Kyngas, H. 4 Hayfield Close, Glen-field, Leicester	Greenhalgh, J., Vanha-nen, L. & Kyngas, H. (1998). Nurse caring behav-iors. *Journal of Advanced Nursing, 27,* 927–932.	Caring behav-iors and how they related to nurses practice in psychiatric and general nurses' views	CARE-Q question-naire with free-choice format **(Interna-tional use of tool: Fin-land)**	n = 69 nurses from psy-chiatric hospital in Northern Finland; n = 49 nurses from gen-eral hospi-tal, Northern Finland	Larson (1984)	Caring behav-iors from Lar-son (1984)	

Master Matrix Blueprint for All Instruments for Measuring Caring *(continued)*

Instrument	Author Contact Address	Publication Citation Source	Developed to Measure	Instrument Description	Participants	Reported Validity/ Reliability	Conceptual/ Theoretical Basis of Measurement	Latest Citation in Nursing Literature
CARE-Q	Holroyd, E., Yue-kuen, C., Sau-wai, C., Fung-shan, L., & Wai-wan, W. Department of Nursing The Chinese University of Hong Kong	Holroyd, E., Yue-kuen, C., Sau-wai, C., Fung-shan, L. & Wai-wan, W. (1998). *Journal of Advanced Nursing, 28*(6), 1289–1294.	Nursing caring behaviors in an acute care setting	**International Chinese version of CARE-Q** with five-point Likert-type fixed rating measure	n = 29 inpatients from acute public hospital in Hong Kong	Face and content validity based upon Larson (1984) Reliability in test-retest study-item ranking consistency for top 5 items No Chinese version reliability or validity tested	Nurse caring behaviors; Larson (1984)	

(continued)

Master Matrix Blueprint for All Instruments for Measuring Caring *(continued)*

Instrument	Author Contact Address	Publication Citation Source	Developed to Measure	Instrument Description	Participants	Reported Validity/ Reliability	Conceptual/ Theoretical Basis of Measurement	Latest Citation in Nursing Literature
CARE-Q (Caring Assessment Instrument)	Larsson, G., Peterson, V. W., Lampic, C., von Essen, L., Sjoden, P. Centre for Caring Sciences, Uppsals University, SWEDEN *Louise-von.essen@ ccs.uu.se*	Larsson, G., Peterson, V. W., Lampic, C., von Essen, L., Sjoden, P. (1998). Cancer patient and staff ratings of the importance of caring behaviors and their relation to patient anxiety and depression. *Journal of Advanced Nursing, 27,* 855–864.	Caring behaviors and patient levels of anxiety and depression in cancer patients	CARE-Q **International version (Swedish)** Larson (1984) von Essen et al. (1994)	n = 53 patients with cancer diagnosis n = 62 staff from 3 units Swedish hospital in Uppsala	Refers to reliability/ validity von Essen & Sjoden (1993)	Caring behaviors original Larson (1994)	**This citation (1998) latest publication of Swedish version of CARE-Q research**

277

Master Matrix Blueprint for All Instruments for Measuring Caring   *(continued)*

Instrument	Author Contact Address	Publication Citation Source	Developed to Measure	Instrument Description	Participants	Reported Validity/ Reliability	Conceptual/ Theoretical Basis of Measurement	Latest Citation in Nursing Literature
CARE/ SATISFAC- TION Question- naire (CARE/ SAT) (1993) RE- VISION OF CARE-Q	Patricia Lar- son, DNS., RN (UCSF) Sandra Fer- ketich, PhD, RN Dean, U. of New Mexico	Larson, P. & Ferketich, S. (1993). Pa- tients' satis- faction with nurses' car- ing during hospitaliza- tion. *Western Journal of Nursing Re- search, 15*(6), 690–707.	Patient satis- faction of nursing care	Descriptive correlational study Visual Ana- log scale adapted from CARE-Q; 29 items	n = 268 pa- tients	Cronbach's alpha Construct and concur- rent validity reported Factor analy- sis = 3 factors to account for variance	Original work of Lar- son, with adaptation	

Master Matrix Blueprint for All Instruments for Measuring Caring *(continued)*

Instrument and Year Developed	Author Contact Address	Year Published Source Citation	Developed to Measure	Instrument Description	Participants	Reported Reliability/ Validity	Conceptual-Theoretical Basis	Latest Citation to Date
Caring Behavior Inventory (CBI) 1981, 1983, 1986	Zane Wolf, RN, PhD, La Salle University School of Nursing, 1900 West Olney Ave. Philadelphia, PA 19141 *wolf@lasalle.edu* Ph: (215) 951-1432 Fax: (215) 951-1896	Wolf, Z. R. (1986). The caring concept & nurse identified caring behaviors. *Topics in Clinical Nursing,* 8(2), 84–93.	Words, phrases in nursing literature that represent caring (attitudes and actions)	42 final items, derived from 75 original words/ phrases 4-point Likert Scale; easy to use; brief to administer	Nurses n = 97	Content validity from literature sources	Strongly informed by Watson theory (1988); refers to transpersonal and 10 carative factors	Wolf et al. (1998). Research Utilization: Relationship between nurse caring and patient satisfaction. *MEDSURG Nursing,* 7(2), 99–105.

(continued)

Master Matrix Blueprint for All Instruments for Measuring Caring *(continued)*

Instrument and Year Developed	Author Contact Address	Year Published Source Citation	Developed to Measure	Instrument Description	Participants	Reported Reliability/ Validity	Conceptual-Theoretical Basis	Latest Citation to Date
								Swan, B. A. (1998). Research utilization. Postoperative nursing care contributions to symptom distress and functional status after ambulatory surgery. *Medsurg. Nursing,* 7(3), 148–151.

Master Matrix Blueprint for All Instruments for Measuring Caring *(continued)*

Instrument and Year Developed	Author Contact Address	Year Published Source Citation	Developed to Measure	Instrument Description	Participants	Reported Reliability/ Validity	Conceptual-Theoretical Basis	Latest Citation to Date
CBI revised 1986, 1994	Zane Wolf (above)	Wolf, Z., et al. (1994). Dimensions of nurse caring. *Image: Journal of Nursing Scholarship*, 26(2), 107–111.	Process of caring	4-point Likert (suggested to use 7-point Likert) 42-items based on words/ phrases	Nurses n = 278 Patients n = 263	Test-retest reliability 0.96 on 278 nurses; content & construct validity— expert panel; factor analysis: 5 items; 42 items	Watson's theory; transpersonal dimensions	See Wolf et al. (1998)

(continued)

Master Matrix Blueprint for All Instruments for Measuring Caring *(continued)*

Instrument and Year Developed	Author Contact Address	Year Published Source Citation	Developed to Measure	Instrument Description	Participants	Reported Reliability/ Validity	Conceptual-Theoretical Basis	Latest Citation to Date
CBI 1998 Retesting	Dr. Zane Wolf See above	Wolf et al. (1998). Relationship between nurse caring and patient satisfaction. *MEDSURG Nursing, 7*(2), 99–105.	Retesting with adult patients caring process and actions	Original instrument with 6-point Likert scale	n = 335 Adult hospitalized medical surgical patients	Overall Cronbach's alpha 0.98; reading level reported at 5.9 and reading ease at 60.7.	Watson's Transpersonal Caring Theory	Wolf et al. (1998). Relationship between nurse caring and patient satisfaction. *MEDSURG Nursing, 7*(2), 99–105.

Master Matrix Blueprint for All Instruments for Measuring Caring *(continued)*

Instrument/ Year Developed	Author Contact Address	Year Published/ Source Citation	Developed to Measure	Instrument Description	Participants	Reported Reliability/ Validity	Theoretical- Conceptual Basis	Latest Citation in Nursing Literature
Caring Behavior Assessment Instrument (CBA) 1988	Sherill Cronin, RN, PhD & Barbara Harrison, MEd., RN, Lansing School of Nursing, Bellarmine Nursing, Bellarmine College, Newburg Road, Louisville, KY 40205-0671 *scronin@ bellarmine. edu*	Cronin, S., & Harrison, B. (1988). Importance of nurse caring behaviors as perceived by patients after myocardial infarction. *Heart and Lung, 17(4),* 374–380.	Patient's perception of nurse caring behaviors; explicitly attempts to address process	63 items 7 subscales 5-point Likert rating	Post-myocardial infarction patients n = 22	Cronbach's alpha established; face and content validity obtained	Watson's Theory of caring and 10 carative factors in theory	Manogin, T. W., Bechtel, G., & Rami, R. (2000). Caring behaviors by nurses: Women's perceptions during childbirth. *JOGNN, 29(2),* 153–157.

(continued)

Master Matrix Blueprint for All Instruments for Measuring Caring *(continued)*

Instrument/ Year Developed	Author Contact Address	Year Published/ Source Citation	Developed to Measure	Instrument Description	Participants	Reported Reliability/ Validity	Theoretical-Conceptual Basis	Latest Citation in Nursing Literature
CBA (further testing)	Margaret Helene Stanfield, PhD Texas Women's University	Stanfield, M. H. (1991). Watson's caring theory and instrument development. *Dissertation Abstracts International,* 52(8), 4128–B. Order No. DA 9203096. 158 pp.	Patients' perceptions of caring	63 items 7 subscales, based on Watson's carative factors	N = 104 adult hospitalized patients medical-surgical unit	Alpha for whole instrument .9566; subscales, alpha .7825–.8867; construct validity established with factor analysis	Watson's theory of caring and 10 carative factors	

Master Matrix Blueprint for All Instruments for Measuring Caring *(continued)*

Instrument/ Year Developed	Author Contact Address	Year Published/ Source Citation	Developed to Measure	Instrument Description	Participants	Reported Reliability/ Validity	Theoretical-Conceptual Basis	Latest Citation in Nursing Literature
CBA (revised) 1993	Elizabeth Parsons, MSN, RN, Carolyn Kee, PhD, RN, Crawford, W. Long Hospital of Emory University, Atlanta, Georgia	Parson, E., Kee, C., et al. (1993). Perioperative Nursing Caring Behaviors. *AORN Journal, 57*(5), 1106–1114.	Patients' perceptions of nurse caring behaviors	63 items, 5-point Likert, 7 subscales (revised original CBA)	Post surgery patients (short stay) n = 19	Based upon Cronin & Harrison (1988)	Watson caring theory and 10 carative factors	ditto

(continued)

Master Matrix Blueprint for All Instruments for Measuring Caring *(continued)*

Instrument/ Year Developed	Author Contact Address	Year Published/ Source Citation	Developed to Measure	Instrument Description	Participants	Reported Reliability/ Validity	Theoretical- Conceptual Basis	Latest Citation in Nursing Literature
CBA (revised) 1993	Kathleen Huggins, MSN, RN, William Gandy, EdD, & Catherine Kohut Baptist Memorial Hospital, Memphis, TN	Huggins, K., Gandy, W., & Kohut, C. (1993). Emergency department patient perceptions of nurse caring behaviors. *Heart and Lung,* 22(4), L356–364.	Patients' perceptions of nurse caring behaviors	Modified for phone survey & emergency patients 65 items; 4-point ordinal; 6 subscales	Emergency Patients n = 288	Original reports of Cronin & Harrison (1988)	Watson theory/10 carative factors	ditto

Master Matrix Blueprint for All Instruments for Measuring Caring *(continued)*

Instrument/ Year Developed	Author Contact Address	Year Published/ Source Citation	Developed to Measure	Instrument Description	Participants	Reported Reliability/ Validity	Theoretical-Conceptual Basis	Latest Citation in Nursing Literature
CBA original	Iris L. Mullins Auburn University, School of Nursing, Auburn, AL	Mullins, I. L. (1996). Nurse caring behaviors for persons with AIDS/HIV. *Applied Nursing Research*, 9(1), 18–23.	Identify caring behaviors desired by patients with AIDS/HIV	63 nurse caring behaviors, open-ended question at end of CBA	n = 46 from AIDS outreach groups and AIDS support groups; 4 geographical areas in SE USA	Reliability and validity from Cronin & Harrison (1988)	Watson theory and carative factors as rationale for selecting CBA	ditto

(continued)

287

Master Matrix Blueprint for All Instruments for Measuring Caring   *(continued)*

Instrument/Year Developed	Author Contact Address	Year Published/Source Citation	Developed to Measure	Instrument Description	Participants	Reported Reliability/Validity	Theoretical-Conceptual Basis	Latest Citation in Nursing Literature
CBA Original Cronin & Harrison version	Schultz, C. Bridgham, M. E., Smith, & D. Higgins: Schultz, RN, PhD, nurse researcher, Maine Medical Center (MMC); Bridgham, RN, BSN Head Nurse Maternity Unit, Maine Medical Center; Mary Smith, RN, BSN, Assistant Head Nurse, Maternity, MMC; Diane Higgins, RN, BSN Staff Nurse MCC	Schultz, A. A., Bridgham, C., Smith, M. E., & Higgins, D. (1998). Perceptions of caring. Comparison of antepartum and postpartum patients. *Clinical Nursing Research, 7,* 363–378.	Describe and compare similarities and differences in the perceptions of caring behaviors between antepartum patients and short-term postpartum patients	CBA as developed by Cronin and Harrison (1988) 63 caring behaviors; 5-point Likert scale	n = 42 convenience sample of antepartum and short-term postpartum patients	Reports additional test of reliability; .71–.88 for subscales; alpha of .93 for total scale	Watson's theory; carative factors	ditto

Master Matrix Blueprint for All Instruments for Measuring Caring *(continued)*

Instrument/ Year Developed	Author Contact Address	Year Published/ Source Citation	Developed to Measure	Instrument Description	Participants	Reported Reliability/ Validity	Theoretical- Conceptual Basis	Latest Citation in Nursing Literature
CBA Original	B. Marini, RN, MSN Educator, Continuing Education, Department of Nursing & Allied Health, Bucks County Community College Newtown, PA 705 Darley Circle, New Hope, PA 18938	Marini, B. (1999). Institutionalized older adults' perceptions of nurse caring behaviors. *Journal of Gerontological Nursing, 25*(5), 11–16.	Perceptions of caring from older adults, institutionalized	CBA with 64 nurse caring behaviors, with 7 subscales; plus 1 open-ended question "Is there anything else that nurses do to make you feel cared for or about?"	21 residents in long-term care, assisted-living facility	Additional correlations established on subscales by gender; highest range 0.89 for women; 0.85 for men	Watson's theory; carative factors	ditto

(continued)

Master Matrix Blueprint for All Instruments for Measuring Caring (continued)

Instrument/ Year Developed	Author Contact Address	Year Published/ Source Citation	Developed to Measure	Instrument Description	Participants	Reported Reliability/ Validity	Theoretical-Conceptual Basis	Latest Citation in Nursing Literature
CBA Original	S. Gay, RN, MSN Staff Nurse; Intensive Care Unit St. Francis Hospital, Beech Grove, Indiana	Gay, S. (1999). Meeting cardiac patients' expectations of caring. *Dimensions of Critical Care Nursing, 18*(4), 46–50.	Importance of caring to cardiac patients	CBA 63 items	n = 18 Hospitalized cardiac patients	Report content and face validity with use of panel of experts familiar with Watson's theory; reliability Cronbach's alpha .66–.90.	Watson's caring theory; carative factors	ditto

Master Matrix Blueprint for All Instruments for Measuring Caring *(continued)*

Instrument/ Year Developed	Author Contact Address	Year Published/ Source Citation	Developed to Measure	Instrument Description	Participants	Reported Reliability/ Validity	Theoretical-Conceptual Basis	Latest Citation in Nursing Literature
CBA Original	Toni Winfield Manogin, Assistant Professor; Gregory Bechtel, Professor Graduate Programs Nursing; Janet Rami, Dean, School of Nursing, Southern University School of Nursing, 11161 Paddock Avenue, Baton Rouge, LA 70816 *Gbechtel@ earthlink.net.*	Manogin, T. W., Bechtel, G., & Rami, R. (2000). Caring behaviors by nurses: Women's perceptions during childbirth. *JOGNN,* 29(2), 153–157.	Perception of nurse caring behaviors by women during childbirth	CBA 63 items; 7 subscales	Convenience sample; n = 31 women hospitalized for uncomplicated labor and delivery	Expert panel for content validity; Cronbach's alpha for each of 7 subscales ranged from .66 to .90.	Watson's caring theory and carative factors; earlier work of Cronin & Harrison	ditto

Master Matrix Blueprint for All Instruments for Measuring Caring *(continued)*

Instrument & Year Developed	Author Contact Address	Year Published Source Citation	Developed to Measure	Instrument Description	Participants	Reported Reliability/Validity	Conceptual-Theoretical Basis of Measurement	Latest Citations in Nursing Literature
Caring Behaviors of Nurses Scale (CBNS) Hinds 1985, 1988	Pamela S. Hinds, RN, PhD, CS Director of Nursing Research, St. Jude Children's Research Hospital, 332 North Lauderdale, Memphis, TN 38105 *Pam.Hinds@stjude.org*	Hinds, P. S. (1988). The relationship of nurses' caring behaviors with hopefulness and health care outcomes in adolescents. *Archives of Psychiatric Nursing, 2*(1), 21–29.	Caring behaviors of nurses within inter-subjective human relationship	Inductively based 22-item visual analogue scale, with possible range of 0 to 100 points; highest score, indicating perception of being more cared for by nurse	n = 25 Adolescent inpatients on substance abuse treatment unit in SW	Reported to have face and content validity, form equivalence, and internal consistency (Hinds, 1985); with adolescent study (1988) Cronbach's alpha of 0.86 for two data collection points; pragmatic content analysis and semantic content analysis achieved pre-established criterion levels of .8 or higher across the data collection points inter-coder reliability, stability	Existential-Humanistic Nursing (Paterson & Zderad) inter-subjective relationship of caring	Hinds, 1988

Master Matrix Blueprint for All Instruments for Measuring Caring *(continued)*

Instrument & Year Developed	Author Contact Address	Year Published Source Citation	Developed to Measure	Instrument Description	Participants	Reported Reliability/ Validity	Conceptual-Theoretical Basis of Measurement	Latest Citation of Instrument
Professional Caring Behaviors Horner, 1989, 1991	Sharon D. Horner, PhD, RN, University of Texas at Austin, 1700 Red River, Austin, TX 78701-1499 s.horner@mail.utexas.edu	Personal communication only (Harrison, 1995 publication, see below)	Perceptions of nurse caring behaviors	4 open-ended questions Two Forms (A & B), 28 items each	Patients n = 356	Test-retest .81 Cronbach's alpha .92 & .94 Pearson r .001	None stated, but refers to general caring theory literature	Harrison, E. (1995) Nurse caring: The new health care paradigm. *Journal of Nursing Care Quality*, 9(4), 14–23.

Master Matrix Blueprint for All Instruments for Measuring Caring *(continued)*

Instrument & Year Developed	Author Contact Address	Year Published Source Citation	Developed to Measure	Instrument Description	Participants	Reported Reliability/ Validity	Conceptual-Theoretical Basis of Measurement	Latest Citation of Instrument
Professional Caring Behaviors	Elizabeth Harrison, MS, RN. Staff Nurse IV, Department of Nursing, St. Joseph's Hospital, Milwaukee, Wisconsin	Harrison, E. (1995). Nurse caring: The new health care paradigm. *Journal of Nursing Care Quality, 9*(4), 14–23.	Perceptions of nursing caring behaviors of families and nurses of inpatient hospice clients	28 items of 2 forms: A & B; 4-point Likert scale	Nurses (inpatient hospice) n = 16 Family members of hospice patients n = 15	Content validity Test-retest reliability Cronbach's alpha (See Horner above)	See above Concern with families' perception of nurse caring	ditto

Master Matrix Blueprint for All Instruments for Measuring Caring *(continued)*

Instrument & Year Developed	Author Contact Address	Year Published and Source Citation	Developed to Measure	Instrument Description	Participants	Reported Reliability/Validity	Conceptual-Theoretical Basis of Measurement	Latest Citation in Nursing Literature
Nyberg Caring Attributes Scale (CAS) 1989, 1990	Jan Nyberg, RN, PhD, 13502 W. 63rd Place, Arvada, Colorado 80004 303-425-1219 jannyberg7 @aol.com	Nyberg, J. (1990). The effects of care and economics on nursing practice. *Journal of Nursing Administration*, 20(5), 13–18.	Caring attributes of nurses—more subjective human element, than behaviors	20 items, on five-point Likert scale; 4 separate rating scales on items	n = 135 nurses from random sample mailing of questionnaire	Cronbach's alpha reported at: .87–.98. No discussion of construct or content validity—except use of theory factors, previously tested (Cronin & Harrison, 1988)	Draws directly from caring theory literature, specific items from Watson's caritative factors; others from Noddings, Gaut, Mayeroff	Nyberg, J. (1990). The effects of care and economics on nursing practice. *Journal of Nursing Administration*, 20(5), 13–18.

Master Matrix Blueprint for All Instruments for Measuring Caring *(continued)*

Instrument & Year Developed	Author & Contact Address	Publication Source Citation	Developed to Measure	Instrument Description	Participants	Reported Reliability/ Validity	Conceptual-Theoretical Basis of Measurement	Latest Citation in Nursing Literature
Caring Ability Inventory (CAI)	Ngozi O. Nkongho, RN, PhD Assistant Professor, Lehman College, Department of Nursing, The City University of New York, New York, NY Ph: 718.960.8794 *ngozi@alpha. lehman.cuny. edu*	Nkongho, N. (1990). The Caring Ability Inventory. In *Measurement of Nursing Outcomes. Vol. 4*, O. L. Strickland & C. R. Waltz (Eds.). New York: Springer. 3–13; 14–16.	Ones' ability to care (when involved in relationship)	Self-administered 7-point Likert; 47 items; 3 major factors: knowing, courage, patience; measured with subscales	n = 462 college students, varied majors; n = 75 nurses (attending professional conference)	Cronbach's alpha for each factor (.71–.84 range) Factor Analysis for collapsing items Test-Retest $r = .64–.80$ range content validity with experts; construct validity between group discrimination and correlation with Tennessee Self-Concept Scale	General review of caring theory literature; specific development informed by Mayeroff's eight critical elements of caring	Nkongho, N. (1990). The Caring Ability Inventory. In *Measurement of Nursing Outcomes. Vol. 4*. O. L. Strickland & C. R. Waltz (Eds.) New York: Springer. 3–13; 14–16. Cavanaugh, S., & Simmons, P. (1997). Evaluation of a school climate for assessing af-

Master Matrix Blueprint for All Instruments for Measuring Caring *(continued)*

Instrument & Year Developed	Author & Contact Address	Publication Source Citation	Developed to Measure	Instrument Description	Participants	Reported Reliability/ Validity	Conceptual-Theoretical Basis of Measurement	Latest Citation in Nursing Literature
								fective objectives in health professional education. *Evaluation and the Health Professions, 20(4),* 455–478. Simmons, P. R., & Cavanaugh, S. H. (2000). Relationships among student and graduate caring ability and professional school climate. *Journal of Professional Nursing, 16(2),* 76–83.

297

Master Matrix Blueprint for All Instruments for Measuring Caring *(continued)*

Instrument and Year Developed	Author & Contact Address	Publication Source Citation	Developed to Measure	Instrument Description	Participants	Reported Reliability/ Validity	Conceptual-Theoretical Basis of Measurement	Latest Citation in Nursing Literature
Caring Behaviors Checklist (CBC)	Anna McDaniel, RN, CS, MA. Last Contact Address: Assistant Professor of Nursing Education, Division of Nursing, Indiana Wesleyan University, Marion, Indiana **(unable to obtain current contact address)**	McDaniel, A. M. (1990). The caring process in nursing: Two instruments for measuring caring behaviors. In *Measurement of Nursing Outcomes.* Strickland, O., & Waltz, C. (Eds.). New York: Springer: 17–27.	Caring process (external observable)	12 items of observable caring behaviors; dichotomous scoring of each item by trained observer(s)	Junior Nursing Student—patient interactions n = not given	Interrater reliability, 92 overall on 12 items; Content Validity Index (CVI) .80	Informed by philosophical views in general caring literature; interest in *caring about* as well as *caring for,* guided instrument development	McDaniel, A. M. (1990). The caring process in nursing: Two instruments for measuring caring behaviors. In *Measurement of Nursing Outcomes.* Strickland, O., & Waltz, C. (Eds.) New York: Springer.

(continued)

Master Matrix Blueprint for All Instruments for Measuring Caring *(continued)*

Instrument and Year Developed	Author & Contact Address	Publication Source Citation	Developed to Measure	Instrument Description	Participants	Reported Reliability/ Validity	Conceptual-Theoretical Basis of Measurement	Latest Citation in Nursing Literature
Client Perception of Caring Scale (CPC)	McDaniel, A. M. (see above)	Citation above	Clients' perception of nurse caring (detect both caring and non-caring behaviors as perceived by clients)	Designed to be used with CBC in hospital setting 10 items rated on 6-point scale; Scores range from 10–60	Number of participants not given; junior-level nursing students in BS nursing program	Content Validity 1.00 using CVI Alpha .81 reliability; item to total correlation .41 Construct validity not significant after correction with Empathy scale	General caring theory literature; Conceptual model of caring process developed to guide instrument	McDaniel, A. M. (1990). The caring process in nursing: Two instruments for measuring caring behaviors. In *Measurement of Nursing Outcomes.* Strickland, O., & Waltz, C. (Eds.) New York: Springer.

Master Matrix Blueprint for All Instruments for Measuring Caring *(continued)*

Instrument and Year Developed	Author & Contact Address	Year Publication Source Citation	Developed to Measure	Instrument Description	Participants	Reported Reliability/ Validity	Conceptual-Theoretical Basis of Measurement	Latest Citation in Nursing Literature
Caring Assessment Tool (CAT) Duffy 1990, 1992	Duffy, J. DNS Associate Professor of Nursing, Catholic University of America, Washington, DC 20064 202-319 6466 *Duffy@cua.edu*	Duffy, J. (1992). The impact of nurse caring on patient outcomes. In D. Gaut (Ed.), *The Presence of Caring in Nursing.* New York: NLN:113–136.	Patients' perception of nurse caring behaviors	100 items 5-point Likert	Medical-Surgical Patients n = 86	Internal consistency, test-retest reliability established; content validity reported in Duffy, 1990, dissertation work	Watson's theory of human caring; 10 carative factors	Duffy, J. (1993). Caring behaviors of nurse managers: Relationship to staff nurse satisfaction & retention. In Gaut, D., A *Global Agenda for Caring.* New York: NLN:365–378.

(continued)

Master Matrix Blueprint for All Instruments for Measuring Caring *(continued)*

Instrument and Year Developed	Author & Contact Address	Year Publication Source Citation	Developed to Measure	Instrument Description	Participants	Reported Reliability/ Validity	Conceptual-Theoretical Basis of Measurement	Latest Citation in Nursing Literature
Caring Assessment Tool (Administrator Form) CAT-admin Duffy (1992, 1993)	See above	Duffy, J. (1993). Caring behaviors of nurse managers: Relationship to staff nurse satisfaction & retention. In Gaut, D., *A Global Agenda for Caring*. New York: NLN:365–378.	CAT-admin. Modified for nurses perception of managers' caring behaviors; Relationship between staff nurse satisfaction & nurse managers' caring	94 items 5-point Likert	Nurses n = 56	See CAT, above & contact author	Watson's Theory and carative factors	See above
Caring Assessment Tool CAT-edu, Educational form of CAT Duffy, 2001	Duffy, 2001 See above	No publication source citation at this time	Educational version of CAT, focus on assessing students' perceptions of caring	5-point Likert scale; 95 items	n = 71 nursing students; baccalaureate and master's level	Earlier validity established; new Reliability on CAT-edu alpha = .9812	Original theory and conceptual basis: Watson Caring theory and Carative Factors	No publication to date on CAT-edu

Master Matrix Blueprint for All Instruments for Measuring Caring *(continued)*

Instrument & Year Developed	Author and Contact Information	Publication Source Citation	Developed to Measure	Instrument Description	Participants	Reported Validity/ Reliability	Conceptual-Theoretical Basis of Measurement	Latest Citation in Nursing Literature
Peer Group Caring Interaction Scale (PCGIS) 1993, 1998	Linda Hughes Associate Professor Nursing, University of Texas Medical Branch, 301 University Blvd., Galveston, Texas 77555-1029 Ph: 409-772-8255 FAX 409 772 8323 *lchughes@ utmb.edu*	Hughes, L. (1993). Peer group interactions and the student perceived climate for caring. *Journal of Nursing Education, 32*(2), 78–83. Hughes, L. C. (1998). Development of an instrument to measure caring peer group interactions.	Organizational climate of caring perceived among nursing student peer group	16 items; 6-point Likert with 2 subscales: Modeling & Giving Assistance	n = 873 BSN students at 87 NLN accredited, State approved schools of nursing	Cronbach's alpha .91 for each subscale Factor analysis; convergent validity based on positive correlations with the intimacy subscale of the OCDQ and the Peer Group Interaction Scale; Divergent validity based on negative	No formal conceptual-theoretical framework identified; but indirectly informed by caring literature and caring theories as well as educational theories, e.g. Noddings (1984) and Bevis (Bevis &	Hughes, L. C., Kosowski, M. M., Grams, K. & Wilson, C. (1998). Caring interactions among nursing students: A descriptive comparison of two associate degree nursing programs. *Nursing Outlook, 4*(4), 176–181. (Development of instrument,

(continued)

Master Matrix Blueprint for All Instruments for Measuring Caring *(continued)*

Instrument & Year Developed	Author and Contact Information	Publication Source Citation	Developed to Measure	Instrument Description	Participants	Reported Validity/ Reliability	Conceptual-Theoretical Basis of Measurement	Latest Citation in Nursing Literature
		correlation with the *Journal of Nursing Education*, 37(5), 202–207.				disengagement subscale of the OCDQ (Hughes, 1998)	Watson, 1989, 2000)	funded by Kansas Health Foundation, Summer Research Award)
Organizational Climate for Caring Questionnaire (OCCQ) Hughes, 1993	Hughes, as above	Hughes, L. (1993). *Relationships among the organizational characteristics of baccalaureate schools of nursing and the student-perceived organizational climate for caring.* Unpublished	Designed to measure student-perceived organizational climate for caring within context of faculty-student interactions	39 items and four subscales: Modeling, Dialogue, Practice, and Confirmation	Junior students enrolled at an accredited BSN school of nursing; Pilot #1: n = 180 students from 20 nursing schools; Pilot #2: n = 363 students from 27 schools;	3 pilot studies; content validity; alpha subscales ranged from .88 to .92; Convergent validity established; Factor analysis yielding four factors: Modeling/ dialogue; Practice,	Noddings' caring ethic and moral development for caring curriculum	Huber, D. I., Maas, M., McCloskey, J., Scherb, C. A., Goode, C. J. & Watson, C. (2000). Evaluating nursing administration instruments. *Journal of Nursing Administration, 30*(5), 251–272. Development

Master Matrix Blueprint for All Instruments for Measuring Caring *(continued)*

Instrument & Year Developed	Author and Contact Information	Publication Source Citation	Developed to Measure	Instrument Description	Participants	Reported Validity/ Reliability	Conceptual-Theoretical Basis of Measurement	Latest Citation in Nursing Literature
		Doctoral Dissertation. The University of Texas at Austin. Hughes, L. A (1992). Faculty-student interactions and the student-perceived climate for caring. *ANS, 14*(3), 60–71.			Pilot #3: n = 853 students from 87 schools	Confirmation, Uncaring Behaviors		of instrument funded by NIH-NINR, Predoctoral Fellowship #1 F31 NR06531

Master Matrix Blueprint for All Instruments for Measuring Caring *(continued)*

Instrument & Year Developed	Author & Contact Address	Year Publication Source Citation	Developed to Measure	Instrument Description	Participants	Reported Reliability/Validity	Conceptual-Theoretical Basis of Measurement	Latest Citation in Nursing Literature
Caring Efficacy Scale 1992, 1995	Carolie Coates, PhD Research & Measurement Consultant, 1441 Snowmass Ct., Boulder, Colorado 80303 303-499-5756 *Coatesc@home.com*	Coates, C. (1997). The Caring Efficacy Scale: Nurses' self-reports of caring in practice settings. *Advanced Practice Nursing Quarterly,* 3(1), 53–59.	Assess conviction or belief in one's ability to express a caring orientation, develop caring relationship with patients	Original 46 items 6-point Likert-type scale Current has 30 items (both self-report and supervisor format) Short Form 12 items	n = 110 nursing students n = 119 alumni n = 117 alumni employers n = 67 clinical supervisors	Cronbach's alpha Form A = .85; Form B = .88; shorter version of Form B = .84 Content validity against Theory/Watson's Carative factors Significant positive correlation between Clinical Evaluation Tool (alpha .85 and .95) and CES	Bandura's social psychology Self Efficacy Scale and Watson's Caring Theory/10 Carative factors	Coates, C. (1997). The Caring Efficacy Scale: Nurses' self-reports of caring in practice settings. *Advanced Practice Nursing Quarterly,* 3(1), 53–59.

Master Matrix Blueprint for All Instruments for Measuring Caring (continued)

Instrument and Year	Author and Contact Address	Publication Source Citation	Developed to Measure	Instrument Description	Participants	Reported Validity/Reliability	Conceptual-Theoretical Basis of Measurement	Latest Citation in Nursing Literature
Holistic Caring Inventory, Latham, 1988, 1996	Christine Pollack Latham, DNSc., RN, Professor & Dept. Chair, Nursing Department California State University, Fullerton, PO Box 6868, Fullerton, CA 92834-6868 FAX: 714 278 3338 Ph: 714 278 2291 Email: *clatham @fullerton.edu*	Latham, C. P. (1996). Predictors of patient outcomes following interactions with nurses. *Western Journal of Nursing Research, 18(5),* 548–564.	Humanistic caring; patients' perceptions of caring	39-item, Likert-type scale; four-point summation instrument, with 4 caring subscales: physical; interpretive, spiritual, & sensitive	1988 dev. and testing: n = 218 hospitalized patients; 1996: n = 120 acutely ill, hospitalized adults, from 2 medical units of 2 medical centers	Content validity via 2 caring experts; Discriminant validity reported; Cronbach's alpha for 4 subscales: Physical = .90; Interpretive = .89; Spiritual = .91; Sensitive = .90	Psychology theory: Howard (1975) Holistic Dimension of Humanistic Caring Theory	Latham, C. P. (1996). Predictors of patient outcomes following interactions with nurses. *Western Journal of Nursing Research, 18(5),* 548–564. Williams, S. A. (1998). Quality and care: patients' perceptions. *Journal Nursing Care Quality, 12(6),* 18–25.

Master Matrix Blueprint for All Instruments for Measuring Caring *(continued)*

Instrument and Year Developed	Author Contact Address	Year Publication & Source Citation	Developed to Measure	Instrument Description	Participants	Reported Reliability/ Validity	Conceptual-Theoretical Basis of Measurement	Latest Citation in Nursing Literature
Caring Dimensions Inventory (CDI) Watson & Lea, 1997	Roger Watson, PhD, Professor, Department of Nursing, The University of Hull, Cottingham Road, Hull, England HU6 7RX Dr. Amandah (Lea) Hoogbruin, PhD, Nursing Faculty, Kwantlen	Watson, R., Lea, A. (1997). The caring dimensions inventory (CDI): Content validity, reliability and scaling. *Journal of Advanced Nursing, 25,* 87–94.	Perceptions of caring from large sample of nurses	5-point Likert Scale with 41 questions: 25 core questions re: perceptions of caring	n = 1452 Nurses and nursing students	Cronbach's alpha = .91 Mokken Scaling and Spearman's correlation of age; Kruskal-Wallis 1-way ANOVA for male vs. female (p < 0.05) for age and sex differences in perceptions of caring	Empirical approach vs. theoretical basis, although caring theory that supported operationalizing of caring was influential	Lea, A., Watson, R., Deary, I.J. (1998). Caring in Nursing: A Multivariate Analysis. *Journal of Advanced Nursing, 28(3),* 662–671. Lea, A. & Watson, R. (1999). Research in

Master Matrix Blueprint for All Instruments for Measuring Caring *(continued)*

Instrument and Year Developed	Author Contact Address	Year Publication & Source Citation	Developed to Measure	Instrument Description	Participants	Reported Reliability/ Validity	Conceptual-Theoretical Basis of Measurement	Latest Citation in Nursing Literature
	University College, 12666-72nd Avenue, Surrey, BC, CANADA V3W 2M8 *amandah@ interchange. ubc.ca*							brief. Perceptions of caring among nurses: the relationship to clinical area. *Journal of Clinical Nursing, 8*(5), 617–618. Walsh, M. (1999). Nurses and nurse practitioners 1: priorities in care. *Nursing Standard, 13*(24), 38–42.

(continued)

Master Matrix Blueprint for All Instruments for Measuring Caring *(continued)*

Instrument and Year Developed	Author Contact Address	Year Publication & Source Citation	Developed to Measure	Instrument Description	Participants	Reported Reliability/ Validity	Conceptual-Theoretical Basis of Measurement	Latest Citation in Nursing Literature
								Watson, R., Deary, I. J. & Lea, A. (1999). A longitudinal study into the perceptions of caring among nursing students using multivariate analysis of the Caring Dimension Inventory. *Journal of Advanced Nursing, 30,* 1080–1089.

Master Matrix Blueprint for All Instruments for Measuring Caring *(continued)*

Instrument and Year Developed	Author & Contact Information	Source Citation Publication	Developed to Measure	Instrument Description	Participants	Reported Validity/ Reliability	Conceptual-Theoretical Basis of Measurement	Latest Citation in Nursing Literature
Caring attributes professional self-concept—technological influence CAPSTI	David Arthur, Associate Professor, Hong Kong Polytechnic University, Hong Kong, Kowloon, Hong Kong Ph: + 852 2766 6390 Fax: +852 2364 96663 Email: *hsarthur@ inet.polyu. edu.hk*	Arthur, D., Pang, S., Wong, T., Alexander, M. F., et al. (1999). Caring attributes, professional self-concept and technological influences in a sample of registered nurses in eleven countries. *International Journal of Nursing Studies, 36,* 387–396.	Multi-dimensional construct of caring internationally	Uses 3 subscales of caring attributes and 3 subscales of PSCNI—13 items theoretical; 41 items practical; 7 items pedagogical	Total sample 1,957 RNs from 11 countries, e.g., Hong Kong, Australia, Canada, China, Korea, New Zealand, Philippines, Scotland, Singapore, South Africa, Sweden	Cronbach's alpha 0.75 overall; PSCNI = 0.89; TIQ = .75; TISQ = .94; CAQ = .88	Items designed to reflect theoretical, practical, and pedagogical perspectives of caring. Items in 3 categories generated by caring theory literature: e.g., Leininger, Benner, Watson; informed by empirical work of Lea & Watson and Wolf	Arthur, D., et al. (1999). Caring attributes, professional self-concept and technological influences in a sample of registered nurses in eleven countries. *International Journal of Nursing Studies, 36,* 387–396. Arthur, D., Pang, S., & Wong, T. (2001). The effects of technology on the caring attributes of an international sample of nurses. *International Journal of Nursing Studies, 38,* 37–43.

Master Matrix Blueprint for All Instruments for Measuring Caring *(continued)*

Instrument & Year Developed	Author & Contact Information	Year Published & Source Citation	Developed to Measure	Instrument Description	Participants	Reported Reliability/Validity	Conceptual-Theoretical Basis of Measurement	Latest Citation in Nursing Literature
Caring Professional Scale (CPS) Swanson (2000a, b)	Dr. Kristine Swanson Professor of Nursing, Chair of Family and Child Nursing, University of Washington, Box 357262, Seattle, WA 98195 Ph: 206-543-8228 FAX 206-543-6656 *kswanson@u.washington.edu*	Swanson, K. (2000a). Predicting depressive symptoms after miscarriage: A path analysis based on the Lazarus Paradigm. *Journal of Women's Health & Gender-Based Medicine, 9(2),* 191–206.	Consumers rating of health care providers on their practice relationship	14-item, 5-point Likert scale; items derived from Swanson's Caring Theory, and empirical research, that reflects Swanson's empirically derived subcategories: -knowing, -being-with, -doing for, -enabling, and -maintaining belief.	185 women who had experienced miscarriage	Construct and content validity through correlation with Barret-Lennart Relationship Inventory subscale of empathy ($r = .61$, $P < 0.001$); Cronbach's alpha (.74 to .96 advanced clinical practice nurses) (.97 for nurses) & (.96 for physicians)	Swanson's Caring Theory a middle range, empirically derived clinical research-based theory and instrument	Swanson, K. (2000b). A program of research on caring. In M. E. Parker (Ed.), *Nursing Theories and Nursing Practice.* Philadelphia: F. A. Davis NIH, NINR, R29 01899, UW Centre for Women's Health Research, NIH, NINR, P30 NR04001

Master Matrix Blueprint for All Instruments for Measuring Caring *(continued)*

Instrument and Year Developed	Author and Contact Address	Publication Source Citation	Developed to Measure	Instrument Description	Participants	Reported Reliability/ Validity	Conceptual-Theoretical Basis of Measurement	Latest Citation in Nursing Literature
Methodist Health Care System Nurse Caring Instrument (MHCSNCI)	Mary Shepherd, RN, MSN, CNAA Director, Methodist Health Care System, 6565 Fannin Street, Houston, Texas 77030-2707 Ph: 713-790 2531 *MLShepherd@ tmh.tmc.edu* Dr. Gwen Sherwood Professor of Nursing, University of Texas-Houston, Health Sciences Center, School of Nursing, Houston, Texas FAX: 713 500 2026 *gsherwoo@son1. nur.uth.tmc.edu*	Unpublished to date, 2001	Valid and reliable instrument of nurses' caring; to operationalize caring as a core concept in patient satisfaction and outcome-based research on nurses' caring	20-item Likert-type scale; measures dominant components of caring	n = 200 nurses; 21 patients; revised version to sample of n = 369 medical-surgical patients	Intra-Class Correlation 0.98; Construct validity with principal axis factoring with varimax rotation Content validity with staff nurses	Empirically derived from multiple views of caring in the nursing literature; qualitative content analysis	None to date; Two formal research presentations: Shepherd & Sherwood, 1999 Sigma Theta Tau International 35th Biennial convention; Shepherd et al. (2000) International Association for Human Caring Research Conference

Index